Speech Therapy Aphasia Rehabilitation *STAR*

Workbook for Activities of Daily Living (ADLS)

Amanda Anderson M.S. CCC-SLP

Dedication

This workbook is dedicated to Dr. Jodi Dodds, who is an incredible mentor and advocate for people with neurological deficits. As a vascular neurologist, she has amazing compassion for her patients. Thank you for your inspiration to be a better person and to push myself to make a difference for individuals with neurological impairments.

You can access her insightful blog on Facebook by searching for:

The Stroke Blog

Table of Contents:

Introduction

Workbook IV- Activities of Daily Living

This workbook is designed to help with specific tasks that you encounter in your everyday life. The sections are divided up by type of task instead of skill required to complete each task. Some activities require writing, others processing information and following multiple step directions. Others require expressive language skills and many activities require a combination of all of these.

Start with things that are easy for you and work your way up to harder items. The workbook provides guidance to complete real life activities. There are exercises to practice making phone calls and some that require you to use the computer to complete a task. The idea behind this workbook is to combine many skills required for completing day to day activities.

You can pick and choose what areas you want to work on and go from there. Each section provides the opportunity to work on processing skills, receptive language, attention and expressive language skills. Most important, the workbook is designed to build confidence in real life language activities to increase your overall independence.

There is no wrong way to use the workbook. You can use it alone or have a friend or family member go through it with you. You can also use the workbook in a therapy setting. If there are certain areas that are difficult for you, such as writing, naming, or following directions, you can use STAR Workbooks 1-3 to further enhance those skills.

Try to think of this workbook as a jumping off point and use the resources available in it to help you with your everyday life. Practice keeping schedules, writing down appointments and use other compensatory strategies that help you. Each section provides ways to organize a task and use strategies to improve your ability to complete daily challenges on your own. Push yourself to communicate even if it is frustrating and slow at times. The neuroplasticity section explains the benefit of therapy and continued practice to enhance your recovery.

The last section has instructions how to find other resources available to help people with aphasia. There is a network of organizations you can utilize to help support your rehabilitation.

Power of Rehabilitation and Neuroplasticity

Aphasia is a result of damaged brain cells in the language center of your brain. The left hemisphere typically is the dominant hemisphere for both language comprehension and production. Broca's area, located in the left frontal lobe of the brain, controls language production while Wernicke's area lies on the left posterior temporal lobe of the brain and controls language comprehension. All strokes, no matter what kind, damage brain cells. The size and location of the lesion caused by your stroke or brain injury will determine what type of aphasia you have.

Language is a series of messages sent throughout the brain from one neuron to the next until the message is finally understood by your brain and you have selected the appropriate words to answer. When overcoming trauma, the human brain is remarkable and has the capability to reorganize areas of the brain and can even switch language from one hemisphere of the brain to another. The brain can also build new neurons to repair damaged areas. This phenomenon is called neuorplasticity. Basically, the brain has the ability to repair itself after a stroke or brain injury that has damaged brain cells.

After a stroke, the brain is able to repair itself at the neural level by growing new neurons. New neural pathways are formed when one axon grows new nerve endings to reconnect neurons that were severed as a result of damage from a stroke.[1] In other words, new neural pathways are formed to reconnect areas of the brain. Because of

---

[1]HOPES. (June 26, 2010). HOPES Huntington Outreach Project for Education at Stanford. Retrieved from: http://www.stanford.edu/group/hopes/cgi-bin/wordpress/2010/06/neuroplasticity/

neuroplasticity, recovery of both physical and language function is possible through rehabilitation.

New neural pathways do not form spontaneously. The brain needs stimulation at the right pace and timing to facilitate recovery. Research shows that if therapy occurs too quickly it can cause more harm than good.[2] It is ideal to wait a week or two to begin any type of therapy to give the brain time to recover and heal from the initial shock of a stroke.[3] On the opposite spectrum, doing nothing at all can be extremely detrimental. Not only will the area of the brain damaged by the stroke lose all function, but the surrounding areas will begin to atrophy due to lack of stimulation.[4]

How to Facilitate Neuroplasticity

After a stroke or brain injury, from your perspective there isn't anything positive about your situation, but in the world of rehabilitation strokes and brain injuries can be very promising. Neuroplasticity makes recovery possible. It will not be easy. It can take years and a network of support to get back to your premorbid (pre-stroke) self. Unlike progressive diseases like Parkinson's, Multiple Sclerosis or ALS, stroke survivors have the potential to recover. Neurogenesis is the growth of new brain cells and makes recovery of language and physical function possible.[5] There are things you can do to help facilitate neurogenesis. When you wake up every morning remind yourself, "My brain has the ability to repair itself." Use every resource available to you to help your brain recover and regain language function.

---

[2]HOPES. (June 26, 2010). HOPES Huntington Outreach Project for Education at Stanford. Retrieved from:
   http://www.stanford.edu/group/hopes/cgi-bin/wordpress/2010/06/neuroplasticity/

[3]Ibid.

[4]Ibid.

[5]Perlmutter, David MD,. (November 2, 2010). Neurogenesis: How to Change Your Brain. Retrieved from
   http://www.huffingtonpost.com/dr-david-perlmutter-md/neurogenesis-what-it-mean_b_777163.html

It is important to increase your brain's ability to recover from the stroke or brain injury that you just survived. Your goal should be to keep your brain as healthy and receptive to recovery as possible. Multiple research has shown that physical exercise increases the brain's ability to form new neural pathways. One study published in the *Journal of the American Medical Association* found that older adults who participated in regular exercise for 24 weeks had an improvement of 1,800% (that is not a misprint!) in their memory function, language ability, attention and cognitive function compared to a control group of sedentary adults.[6]

Caloric restriction has been shown to increase the brain's ability to grow new brain cells. In 2008, a study of elderly adults found a "significant increase in verbal memory scores after caloric restriction" and no changes in the two control groups who received diets with increased calories and one with no limitations.[7] We all know the benefits of eating a healthy diet full of fruits and vegetables and that is low is saturated fats. Proper nutrition will not only improve your overall health, it can promote further neurogenesis.

DHA and Omega-3 fats also are beneficial in increasing the brain's ability to make new neural pathways. You can find these healthy fats in fish and flaxseed or take them as supplements. While concentrating on what supplements can improve brain function, don't neglect to take your regular multivitamin. Vitamin deficiencies of both zinc and vitamin A have been shown to inhibit normal brain development.[8] Curcumin is the main active ingredient in the spice turmeric, a main ingredients in curry. It is a popular spice in Indian cuisine and also can be taken in supplement form.

---

[6]Perlmutter, David MD,. (November 2, 2010). Neurogenesis: How to Change Your Brain. Retrieved from
http://www.huffingtonpost.com/dr-david-perlmutter-md/neurogenesis-what-it-mean_b_777163.html

[7] Wittea, A,V., Fobkerb, M, Gellnerc R., Knechta, S., Floelad, A. (December, 19, 2008) Caloric restriction improves memory in elderly humans. Retrieved from http://www.pnas.org/content/early/2009/01/26/0808587106

[8]HOPES (July 1, 2011), HOPES Huntington Outreach Project for Education at Stanford. retrieved from
http://www.stanford.edu/group/hopes/cgi-bin/wordpress/2011/07/diet-and-neurogenesis/

Research studies have found curcumin promotes neurogenesis in animals. A vitamin rich, low fat, low calorie diet can be your power fuel for rehabilitation.

How Rehabilitation Works

We know that the brain has the capability to repair itself through the power of neuroplasticity. This doesn't happen overnight and a balance of patient motivation, strong family caregiver and community support and rehabilitation all come together to make recovery possible. How exactly do external forces and stimulus cause the brain to begin to change and expressive and receptive language begin to improve?

Strokes can cause hemiparesis or weakness on one side of the body either in an arm or a leg. With aphasia, the brain has difficulty with word retrieval and sometimes speech can be slurred (dysarthria) or have oral motor planning difficulties (apraxia). Remember, with all of these impairments initially the muscles and nerves in the legs, arms, tongue and face have not been directly damaged. It is in the brain where the damage occurred. By moving the impaired area with assistance of a therapist and using muscles surrounding the weakened area you can stimulate the brain near the damaged area. This stimulation can promote neurogenesis.

Research studies have shown that even minuscule exercises, such as moving your thumb back and forth for 15 minutes, can cause the brain to form new neurons.[9] Aphasia is unique to stroke impairments because there isn't any visible physical impairment. The neural pathways for word retrieval in the language center of the brain have been damaged. To apply the concept of small exercises to aphasia, try something that is easy for you like counting to 10 out loud. Repeat this activity for ten to fifteen

---

[9]Giroux, Holistic Brain Health better living for MS, Parkison's, Dystonia Stroke: Neuroplasticity. retrieved from http://drgiroux.com/neuroplasticity/

minutes. If that is too easy for you, try singing your ABCs for about ten to fifteen minutes, two to three times a day.

Repetition is essential to improving both motor function and expressive language function.[10] Start trying to narrate aloud what you do throughout the day. Even if you have speech therapy 5 times a week an hour a day, that is less than 3% of the week you spend in speech therapy. For best results, you will need to start doing some of the exercises that you do in therapy and make it part of your daily routine. Name items around your room as you use them. After a commercial on TV, say the name of the product that is for sale. Narrate what you do as you do it. Even if you are only able to get a few of the words out it is the attempt that matters, because it stimulates the brain to begin the formation of new neural pathways.

Research studies also show that challenging activities help the recovery of language function. Physical therapists utilize constraint induced movement therapy for stroke survivors. This strategy constrains the unaffected arm of a stroke survivor with hemiparesis, having them to use the arm that had been weakened by the stroke.[11] The weak limb was then isolated to complete daily tasks which produced great results in rehabilitation. This same concept is used in language therapy for aphasia.

Studies have reproduced constraint induced therapy for aphasia. When somebody with aphasia uses the mode of communication that takes the least amount of effort, this is considered similar to using their unaffected arm or leg in physical therapy.[12] It is human nature to avoid frustration and take the path of least resistance.

---

[10]Giroux, Holistic Brain Health better living for MS, Parkison's, Dystonia Stroke: Neuroplasticity. retrieved from http://drgiroux.com/neuroplasticity/

[11] Stroke Connection Magazine (September/October 2004)Constraint induced movement therapy retrieved from http://www.strokeassociation.org/STROKEORG/LifeAfterStroke/RegainingIndependence/PhysicalChallenges/Constraint-Induced-Movement-Therapy_UCM_309798_Article.jsp

[12] Friedemann Pulvermüller, PhD,Bettina Neininger, MA,Thomas Elbert, PhD, Bettina Mohr, PhD, Brigitte Rockstroh, PhD. Peter Koebbel, MA, Edward Taub, PhD, (November 11, 2000). **Constraint-Induced Therapy of Chronic Aphasia After** Stroke. Retrieved from http://stroke.ahajournals.org/content/32/7/1621.full

In aphasia rehabilitation the more communication challenges that are taken on in everyday situations, the better the chances for a fuller recovery.[13] Therapy that incorporates shaping or gradual steps up to difficult tasks, like describing with multiple adjectives, has been shown to have excellent results for individuals who were told they had already reached their maximum post stroke potential.[14] The basis of constraint induced therapy for aphasia is to incorporate the difficult communication tasks into everyday life to achieve the highest levels of expressive language function. Start with the communication you are able to do (even a communication board) and gradually increase the difficulty level.

You would be hard pressed to find any research that showed that less interaction and communication translated into better recovery for somebody with aphasia. The most important thing you can do for yourself is to stay active and talk as much as possible. Challenge yourself to communicate and remember that a frustrating task is one that promotes the formation of new neural pathways.

There are many resources available to help carry over therapy and make recovery part of your life. To be successful, challenge yourself throughout the day, every day. Motivation, family and community support, social interaction, and determination to challenge yourself is the perfect combination for a strong recovery.

You can find more information about resources available for people with aphasia in the nonprofit organization, Aphasia Recovery Connection's *Guide to Living with Aphasia*. All proceeds from the book go to support ARC's mission to end isolation for people with aphasia.

---

[13] ibid.
[14]Ibid

Personal Information:

Practicing writing your personal information.

Name:_____

Birth Date:_____

Age:_____

Location:_____

Name:_____

Birth Date:_____

Age:_____

Location:_____

Personal Information:

Name:_____

Birth Date:_____

Age:_____

Location:_____

Medical History:_____

_____

Name:_____

Birth Date:_____

Age:_____

Location:_____

Medical History:_____

_____

Personal Information:

Name:_____

Phone Number:_____

Cell Number:_____

Address:_____

_____

_____

Email address:_____

Emergency Contact's Name:_____

Emergency Contact's Number:_____

Emergency Contact's Address:_____

_____

_____

_____

Personal Information:

Name:_____

Birth Date:_____

Social Security Number:_____

Address:_____

_____

_____

Phone Number:_____

Cell Number:_____

Spouse: _____

Current Location:_____

_____

Closest Relative_____

Children:_____

Personal Information:

Name:_____

Birth Date:_____

Social Security Number:_____

Address:_____

_____

_____

Phone Number:_____

Cell Number:_____

Spouse:_____

Current Location:_____

_____

Closest Relative:_____

Personal Information:

Name:_____

Mother's Maiden Name_____

Parents' Names:_____

Spouse's Name:_____

In-Law's Names:_____

_____

Children:_____

_____

_____

Grandchildren:_____

_____

_____

Contacts:
Important Phone Numbers

Family Name   Phone Number

_____

_____

_____

_____

_____

_____

_____

_____

_____

_____

Contacts:

Friend   Phone Number

_____

_____

_____

_____

_____

_____

_____

_____

_____

_____

Contacts:
Important Phone Numbers

Doctor   Phone Number

_____

_____

_____

_____

_____

_____

_____

_____

Pharmacy:

_____

_____

_____

Calendars:

Practice filling out the calendars for each month. Add important holidays, events and birthdays. Also, add any upcoming appointments.

January

Month/Year:

Sunday	Monday	Tuesday	Wednesday	Thursday	Friday	Saturday

Fill in a holiday for January.

February

Month/Year:

Sunday	Monday	Tuesday	Wednesday	Thursday	Friday	Saturday

What holiday is February the 14th?

March

Month/Year:

Sunday	Monday	Tuesday	Wednesday	Thursday	Friday	Saturday

What holiday is March 17th?

April

Month/Year:

Sunday	Monday	Tuesday	Wednesday	Thursday	Friday	Saturday

What is school vacation called in April?

May

Month/Year:

Sunday	Monday	Tuesday	Wednesday	Thursday	Friday	Saturday

What holiday weekend is in May?

June

Month/Year:

Sunday	Monday	Tuesday	Wednesday	Thursday	Friday	Saturday

Why is June, special for school children?

July

Month/Year:

Sunday	Monday	Tuesday	Wednesday	Thursday	Friday	Saturday

What does the United States of America celebrate on July 4th?

August

Month/Year:

Sunday	Monday	Tuesday	Wednesday	Thursday	Friday	Saturday

What is the weather like in August?

September

Month/Year:

Sunday	Monday	Tuesday	Wednesday	Thursday	Friday	Saturday

Name a holiday weekend in September.

October

Month/Year:

Sunday	Monday	Tuesday	Wednesday	Thursday	Friday	Saturday

What holiday is at the end of the month in October?

November

Month/Year:

Sunday	Monday	Tuesday	Wednesday	Thursday	Friday	Saturday

Name a holiday in November.

What is Black Friday?

December

Month/Year:

Sunday	Monday	Tuesday	Wednesday	Thursday	Friday	Saturday

Name a holiday in December.

What is the weather like in December?

Holidays:

Draw a line from the clue on the left to the holiday on the right.

Decorated Egg   St. Patrick's Day

Stocking   4th of July

Turkey   Halloween

Leprechaun   Valentine's Day

Abraham Lincoln   Easter

Fireworks   Columbus Day

End of Summer   New Year's Day

Ghosts   Christmas

Flowers and Chocolate   Thanksgiving

Nina, Pinta, Santa Maria   President's Day

Time's Square   Labor Day

Birthdays:

Family: Birth Day

_____   _____

_____   _____

_____   _____

_____   _____

_____   _____

_____   _____

_____   _____

_____   _____

_____   _____

_____   _____

Birthdays:

Friends: Birth Day

_____   _____

_____   _____

_____   _____

_____   _____

_____   _____

_____   _____

_____   _____

_____   _____

_____   _____

_____   _____

Birthdays:

1. Describe a favorite childhood birthday party.

2. What was a favorite toy you had as a child?

3. Name 5 different places you could have a birthday party.

4. Where were you born?

5. What would you need to decorate for a birthday party?

6. What is your favorite kind of birthday cake?

7. Describe a birthday party that you hosted.

8. What was your favorite birthday? Why?

9. What would you buy a 7 year old girl for her birthday?

10. What would you buy a 40 year old man for his birthday?

11. Have you ever had a surprise party?

12. What is the longest someone in your family lived?

Birthdays:

Sequence these steps in the correct order. Write 1-6 next to each step.

Wrap a present

_____put on the bow

_____ get out the scissors, wrapping paper and tape

_____ fold the wrapping paper around the present and tape it.

_____ measure the correct amount of wrapping paper for the box

_____ fold the edges of the paper around the sides of the box and tape.

_____ cut the wrapping paper to fit the present.

Cake Celebration
_____ put the candles on the cake

_____ sing "Happy Birthday"

_____ blow out the candles

_____ take the cake out of refrigerator

_____ light the candles

_____ cut the cake and serve

Holidays:

Sequence the holidays in the correct chronological order

_____ Valentine's Day

_____ New Years Day

_____ Columbus Day

_____ Labor Day

_____ St. Patrick's Day

_____ Mother's Day

_____ Thanksgiving

_____ Father's Day

_____ Memorial Day

_____ President's Day

_____ Easter

_____ Independence Day

_____ Halloween

_____ Christmas

Holidays:

1. Name three religious holidays.

2. Name three holidays where you would take off work.

3. Name a special occasion when you would receive flowers.

4. Name a holiday in Winter.

5. Name a Summer holiday.

6. Name the two holidays that mark the beginning and end of summer.

7. What holiday do children go Trick or Treating?

8. Name holidays that involve candy.

9. Which holidays are sad days?

10. Name 10 holidays in chronological order.

10. Name two holidays you might have a picnic.

11. Name three holidays that most people go to work on.

Week Schedule: Appointments

	Sunday	Monday	Tuesday	Wednesday	Thursday	Friday	Saturday
9 am							
10 am							
11 am							
12 pm							
1 pm							
2 pm							
3 pm							
4 pm							
5 pm							

Write in the events into the week's schedule
1. Breakfast on Wednesday with Linda at 9am.
2. Brunch on Sunday at 11 am with Tom.
3. Bridge game 4 pm on Thursday.
4. Movie with Sam on Saturday
5. Shopping outing Monday at 1 pm.
6. Repair man scheduled for Tuesday at 10 am.

Your Dr.'s office called to remind you of an appointment on Wednesday at 8:30 AM. What event will you need to cancel?

Week Schedule: Appointments

	Sunday	Monday	Tuesday	Wednesday	Thursday	Friday	Saturday
9 am							
10 am							
11 am							
12 pm							
1 pm							
2 pm							
3 pm							
4 pm							
5 pm							

Write the events into the week's schedule

1. Exercise Class Monday and Wednesday at 9 am.
2. Physical Therapy Tuesday and Thursday at 2pm
3. Bingo weekends at 4 pm.
4. Dance class Thursdays at 10am.
5. Cleaning service Friday at 2pm.
6. Book club Monday and Wednesday at 4 pm.

Your friend invited you to breakfast this week at 9 am. What days can you go?

Week Schedule: Appointments

	Sunday	Monday	Tuesday	Wednesday	Thursday	Friday	Saturday
9 am							
10 am							
11 am							
12 pm							
1 pm							
2 pm							
3 pm							
4 pm							
5 pm							

Write in your appointments for the week
1. Monday:Dentist appointment at 2 pm.
2. Tuesday: Hair appointment 3pm.
3. Wednesday: Eye doctor 9 am
4. Friday: Physical with primary care doctor 1 pm.
5. Tuesday: Dentist appointment 9 am.

For your physical you can't eat anything before your appointment. Your friend called and asked to take you to lunch at 11 am. Will you be able to join her? What could you do to solve the problem?

Appointments: Problem solving

You have been feeling light headed lately and are having trouble with your eyes. You are worried about driving to your multiple appointments this week. What are some things you could do to make sure you are able to get to your appointments.

Bus? If so, how do you find the schedule and stops?

Facility Transportation? If so, how could you set this up?

Ask a friend or family member? If so, who? What is their contact info. What appointments should take priority if they can only help with one or two?

Public Transportation Van for people with disabilities? If so, how can you find information about this service?

Home health aid or caregiver? How can you find information about such services?

Volunteer? What organizations do you think could help with this?

Times:
Read out loud the following times:

12:00 PM

2:45 PM

1:15 PM

7:57 AM

2:12 PM

3:30 PM

8:30 AM

9:50 AM

10:00 PM

6:20 PM

6:30 AM

8:50 PM

10:10 AM

11:00 AM

Times:

Read the Following times out loud. Circle the times you are awake.

7:00 AM

11:17 AM

1:20 PM

3:30 AM

4:15 PM

3:35 PM

10:11 AM

1:05 AM

12:00 AM

4:18 PM

9:45 PM

2:20 AM

4:50 AM

5:15 AM

Time:

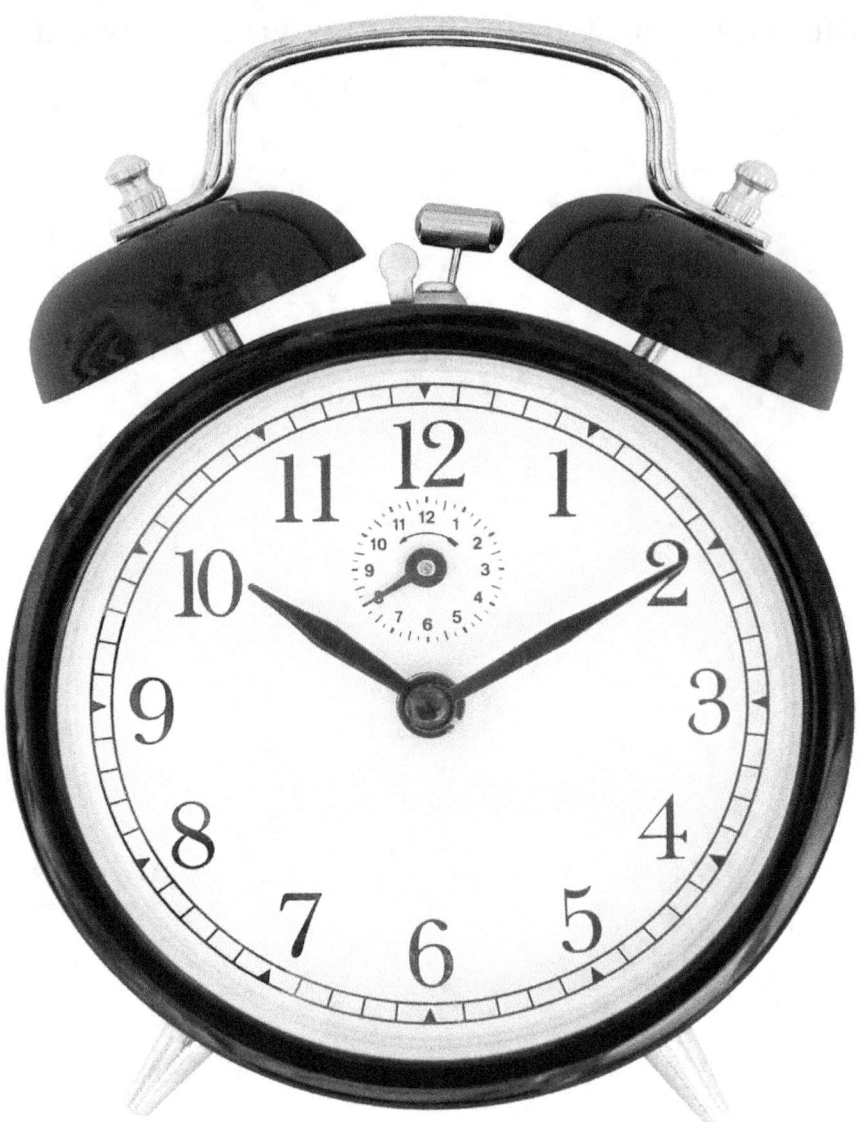

15

1. Read the time on the clock.
2. What type of clock is this?
3. What does the small clock under the 12 count?

15 Source: Sun Ladder CC BY-SA 3.0 via:
http://commons.wikimedia.org/wiki/File:2010-07-20_Black_windup_alarm_clock_face.jpg#mediaviewer/File:2010-07
-20_Black_windup_alarm_clock_face.jpg

Time:

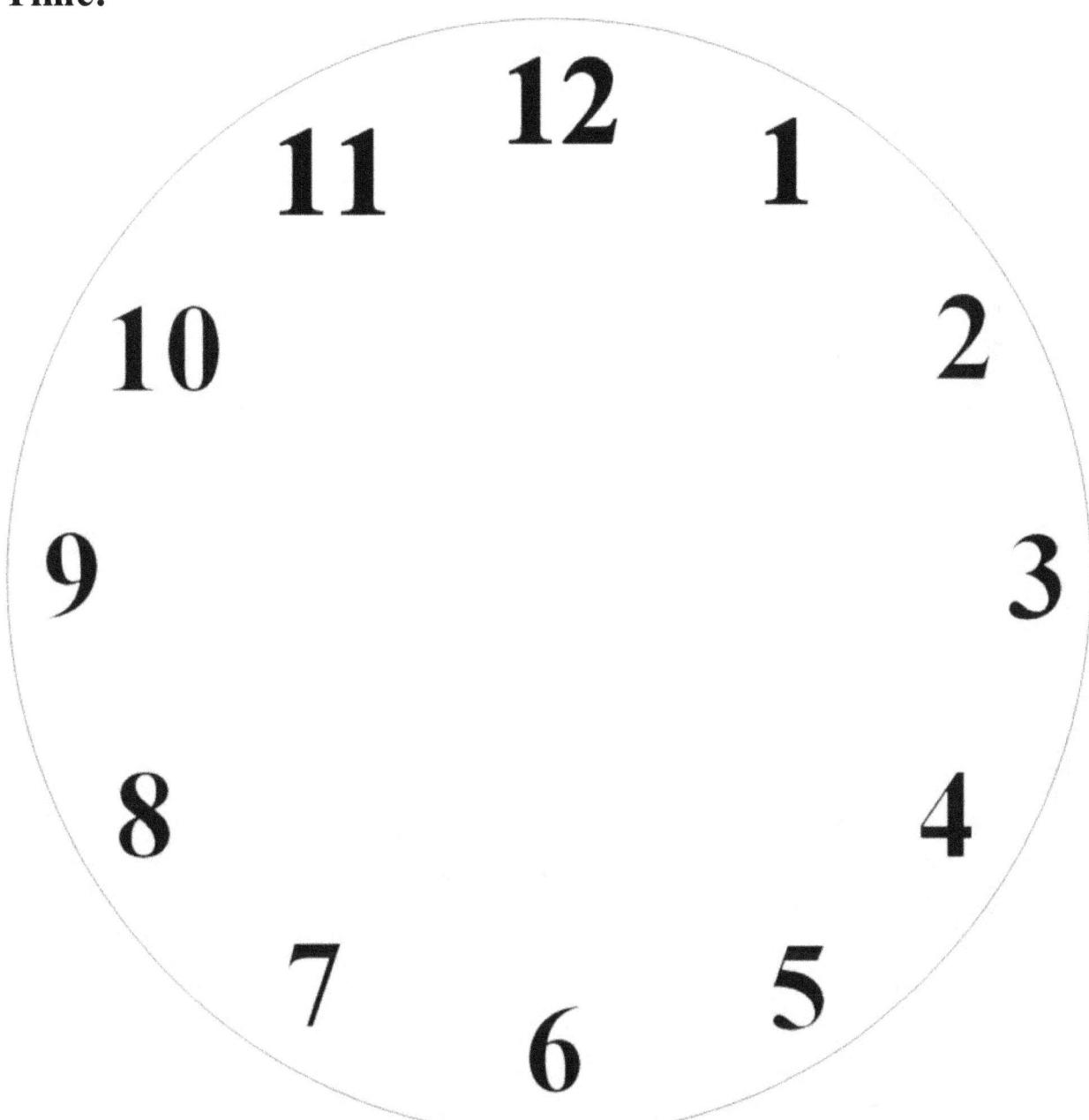

Use items around the house to practice showing the correct times. (A pencil and a crayon can work as the long hand and short hand). Or write in the times with a pencil and then erase. Show the times:

1:15   2:30   5:50   11:25   12:00   4:40

3:30   4:10   2:35   10:55   6:14   8:10

Time: Tell the time on each clock.

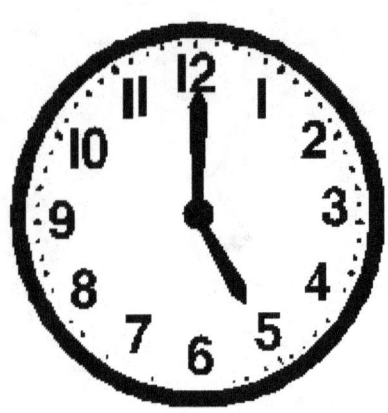

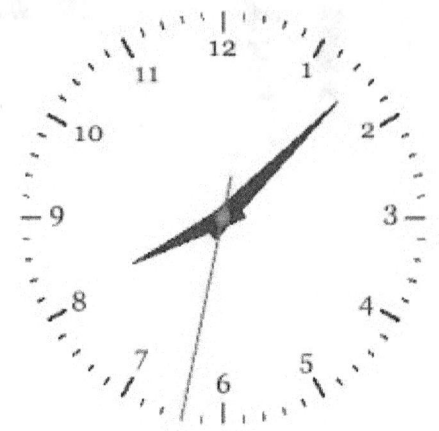

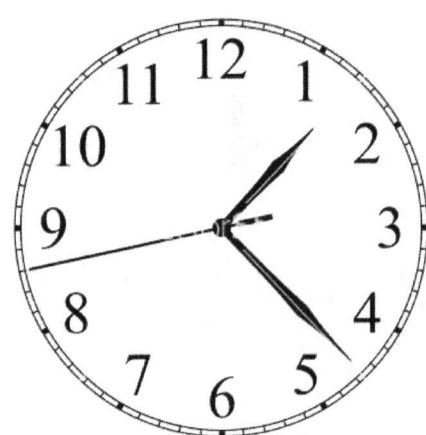

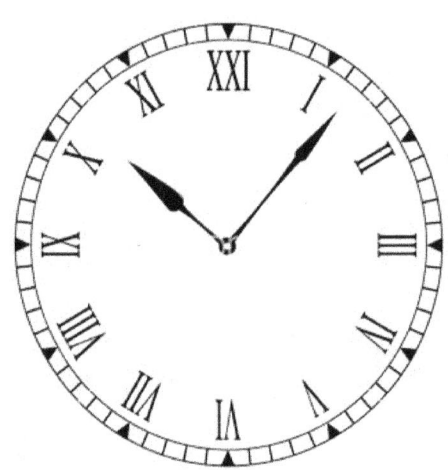

Time: _____

Time: _____

Time: _____

Time: _____

Time:

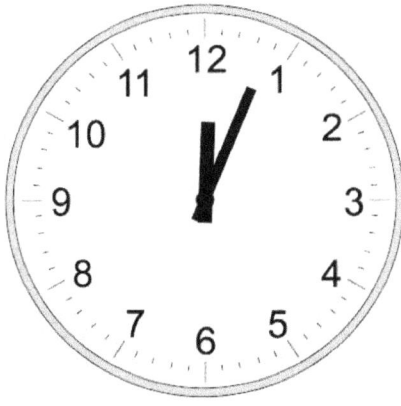

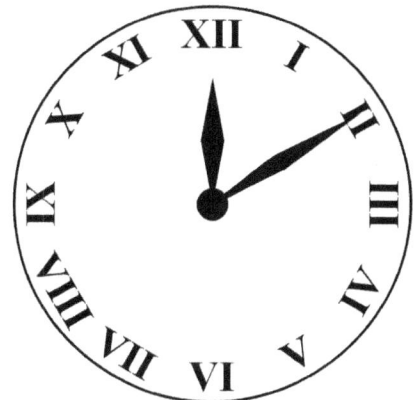

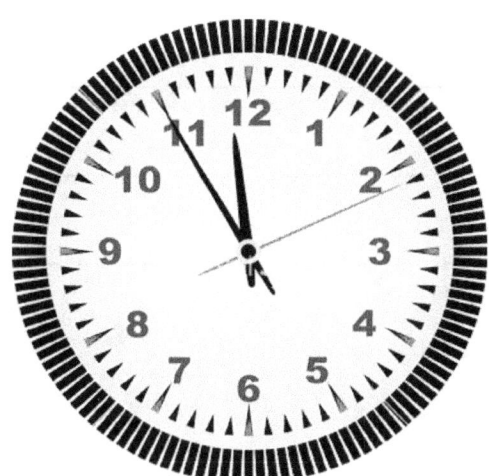

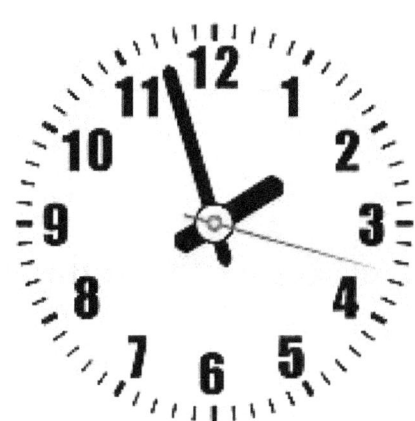

Time:_____   Time:_____

Time:_____   Time:_____

Medications:

Time	Medication
8 AM	
10 AM	
12 PM	
2 PM	
4 PM	
6 PM	
8 PM	
10 PM	

Write the medications on the daily schedule.

Medication List

1. Plavix 75 mg 1x with breakfast
2. Neurotin 1 300 mg pill 3x a day
3. Atenolol 1 100 mg at lunch
4. Ambien 1 pill as needed at bedtime
5. Zoloft 2 pills in the morning

Medications:

Time	Medication
8 AM	
10 AM	
12 PM	
2 PM	
4 PM	
6 PM	
8 PM	
10 PM	

Write the Medications into the daily schedule.

1. Topomax 100mg 2x a day
2. Multivitamin in the morning
3. Noratriptyline 50 mg at bedtime
4. Miralax 1 tablespoon with breakfast as needed

Medications:

Time	Medication
8 AM	
10 AM	
12 PM	
2 PM	
4 PM	
6 PM	
8 PM	
10 PM	

Medications

Write your own medications into the daily schedule

Medication: Problem Solving

1. You are going to be out of town and will need a refill of your heart medication. Insurance will not cover the medication if you refill it before you leave. What can you do to make sure you have your medication when you are away?

2. You are having trouble opening up some of your medication bottles. You don't want to bother your family to open them for you everyday. What are some solutions?

3. You spilled about half of your anxiety medication down the drain by mistake. The pharmacy will not give you an early refill since it is a controlled substance. What can you do?

4. Your doctor recommended that you take 400 mg of Magnesium and fish oil every day. The pills are huge and very hard for you to swallow. What should you do?

5. You called to refill one of your prescriptions but are unable to get to the pharmacy to pick it up. What can you do?

Medication: Medication Problem Solving

These are some tips to help solve some of the problem solving questions.

1 Call your pharmacy in the location where you are going to. If you give them your prescription number they should be able to fill your prescription for you while you are out of town.

2. You could look into getting some of the following medication dispensers.
   - Thirty day pill box. (Your family could fill it up for you but you would only need to ask them once a month)
   - Easy to open pop top bottles
   - Alarm Medication dispenser such as Med-elert (available on amazon for around $80) Some offer alarms and locked medication so you can be positive if you took your medication that day.

3. Most likely you will need to call your doctor to get a new order for your medication. Try to take a picture of the drain with the damaged medication.

4. Ask your pharmacist about chewable or gummy forms of these supplements. You could also take two 200 mg pills which would be smaller.

Medications: Reactions

Your Doctor just started you on a low dose of the medication Lamictal. She gave you the following information to read.

Get emergency medical help if you have any of these signs of an allergic reaction: hives; fever; swollen glands; painful sores in or around your eyes or mouth; difficulty breathing; swelling of your face, lips, tongue, or throat.

Report any new or worsening symptoms to your doctor, such as: mood or behavior changes, depression, anxiety, or if you feel agitated, hostile, restless, hyperactive (mentally or physically), or have thoughts about suicide or hurting yourself.

Lamotrigine may cause severe or life-threatening skin rash, especially in children and in people who take too high of a dose at the start of treatment with lamotrigine. Serious skin rash may also be more likely to occur if you are taking lamotrigine together with valproic acid (Depakene) or divalproex (Depakote). Seek emergency medical attention if you have a fever, sore throat, swelling in your face or tongue, burning in your eyes, skin pain, followed by a red or purple skin rash that spreads (especially in the face or upper body) and causes blistering and peeling.

If you have to stop taking lamotrigine because of a serious skin rash, you may not be able to take it again in the future.

Medications:

Call your doctor at once if you have any of these other serious side effects:

- *the first sign of any skin rash, no matter how mild;*
- *fever, swollen glands, body aches, flu symptoms, headache, neck stiffness, increased sensitivity to light;*
- *easy bruising or bleeding, severe tingling, numbness, pain, muscle weakness;*
- *upper stomach pain, loss of appetite, dark urine, jaundice (yellowing of the skin or eyes);*
- *chest pain, irregular heart rhythm, feeling short of breath;*
- *confusion, nausea and vomiting, swelling, rapid weight gain, urinating less than usual or not at all;*
- *pale skin, feeling light-headed or short of breath, rapid heart rate, trouble concentrating; or*
- *increased seizures or worsening of your bipolar disorder.*

Less serious side effects may include:

- *tremors, dizziness, tired feeling;*
- *blurred vision, double vision;*
- *loss of coordination;*
- *dry mouth, mild nausea, stomach pain, upset stomach;*
- *changes in your menstrual periods;*
- *back pain;*
- *sleep problems (insomnia); or*
- *runny nose, sore throat.*

Medications:

Place a check in the box if the side effect you notice is minor or serious.

Side Effect	Minor	Serious
sore throat		
dry mouth		
skin rash		
confusion		
flu like symptoms		
swelling throat		
burning eyes		
back pain		
fatigue		

If you experience any side effects from a new medication what should you do?

Medication Safety: supplements and vitamins.

Answer the questions based on your own medications.

1. When should you take each medication?
2. Do any medications need to be taken with food?
3. Which medications should be taken at night?
4. What is each medication for?
5. Describe any serious side effects associated with each medication.
6. Are you able to open your medication bottles? If not, who helps you?
7. What should you do with any expired medication?
8. Do you have any children or family members that should not have access to your medications. If so, what safety measures do you have in place?
9. What medications do you take that could be dangerous if you take more than the prescribed dose?
10. What should you do if you take more pills by mistake?
11. Do you have any Ipecac Syrup in case of an emergency? Why would you need it?
12. Your nurse gives you your medication every day. You are used to taking 4 pills, two white pills, one pink and one blue. She gives you 7 pills one day. You tell her it doesn't look like your medication and without checking she tells you to take them. What can you do?

Medication Schedule:

Time of Day	Drug Name	Dose	How many pills?	What is it for?	Prescribing Dr.?
Morning					
Afternoon					
Bedtime					

Medication Schedule:

Time of Day	Drug Name	Dose	How many pills?	What is it for?	Prescribing Dr.?
Morning					
Afternoon					
Bedtime					

Medications:

Select the correct answer(s)

1. You have a bad headache but have already had two glasses of wine. What medication should you avoid?

    a. aspirin

    b. ibuprofen

    c. acetaminophen

    d. sleeping pill

    e. not sure, I'll call the pharmacist to be safe.

2. You can't read the directions on your prescriptions. What can you do?

    a. ask a family member to read them and write it down in larger print.

    b. ask your pharmacist to print out the directions in larger print

    c. use a magnify glass

    d. just try your best to remember

    e. call your doctor

Medication:

3. You keep getting large unsightly bruises since you started taking Plavix. You should:

    a. stop taking the medication

    b. just take a baby aspirin instead

    c. let your doctor know

    d. read the medication side effects

4. You keep forgetting to take your medication in the morning. What can you do?

    a. set a daily alarm

    b. get a medication dispenser

    c. take them whenever you remember

    d. just take them the next day

5. You love to drink grapefruit juice. You remember hearing that grapefruit juice can stop some Medications from working. The paperwork with your new medication doesn't mention anything.

    a. call you pharmacist and ask

    b. call your doctor and ask

    c. read about it on the computer

Medications:

6. Your doctor prescribed 3 refills of your anticoagulant medication. After 3 months, you do not have any refills left. You do not see your Doctor for another 3 weeks. What should you do?

    a. Wait until you see your Doctor to ask about a refill.

    b. Stop taking the medication. You probably only needed it for 3 months.

    c. Ask your pharmacist to call your Dr. to get authorization for more refills.

    d. Call your Dr.'s office to call in another prescription.

7. What can you do in the situation for question 6 if you are unable to verbally ask because of your aphasia.

    a. Show a family member the prescription bottle.

    b. Write down key points like your birthday, Dr.'s name, refill and medication and try on your own to call the pharmacy or Dr's office.

    c. Check to see if you can request refills online.

    d. Bring the prescription bottle to your pharmacy and point to the section that says no refills.

Shopping:

Make a shopping list including 5 fruits, 5 vegetables, 3 snack foods, and two drinks.

1._____

2._____

3._____

4._____

5._____

6._____

7._____

8._____

9._____

10._____

11._____

12._____

13._____

14._____

15._____

Shopping:

Make a shopping list of only foods that will keep at least two months.

1. _____

2. _____

3. _____

4. _____

5. _____

6. _____

7. _____

8. _____

9. _____

10. _____

11. _____

12. _____

13. _____

14. _____

15. _____

16. _____

17. _____

18. _____

19. _____

20. _____

Shopping:

Write a shopping list to make a chicken pot pie, broccoli casserole, garlic bread, red wine and chocolate chip cookies.

1. _____
2. _____
3. _____
4. _____
5. _____
6. _____
7. _____
8. _____
9. _____
10. _____
11. _____
12. _____
13. _____
14. _____
15. _____
16. _____
17. _____
18. _____
19. _____
20. _____

Shopping:

Select the correct answer

1. Circle the vegetable

    a. banana

    b. salmon

    c. apple sauce

    d. carrots

2. Put a line through the items that are not poultry.

    a. chicken

    b. beef

    c. Cornish game hen

    d. pork loin

    e. turkey

3. Put a star next to items you find in the baking aisle.

    a. spices

    b. seafood

    c. flour

    d. sugar

Shopping:

4. Circle the snack items.

    a. lasagna

    b. grapefruit

    c. wheat thins

    d. potato chips

    e. trout

5. Underline the item that you wouldn't find in the dairy aisle.

    a. milk

    b. yogurt

    c. eggs

    d. pretzels

    e. cheese

6. Circle the spices.

    a. cinnamon

    b. salt

    c. sugar

    d. flour

    e. oregano

Shopping:

Name 8 items you would find in the frozen aisle

_____   _____

_____   _____

_____   _____

_____   _____

Name 8 foods you would buy for a dinner party

_____   _____

_____   _____

_____   _____

_____   _____

Name 8 things you would serve at a Super Bowl Party.

_____   _____

_____   _____

_____   _____

_____   _____

Shopping:

Name 8 items at the deli counter.

_____   _____

_____   _____

_____   _____

_____   _____

Name 8 items in the bakery department

_____   _____

_____   _____

_____   _____

_____   _____

Name 8 items in the meat department

_____   _____

_____   _____

_____   _____

_____   _____

Shopping:

Describe the process of shopping at the grocery store using the following words:

1. cart
2. deli
3. coupon
4. check out
5. pay

Describe what you would purchase at the store for Christmas dinner using the following words.

1. table cloth
2. yams
3. ham
4. wine
5. cake

What do you like about the grocery store where you shop?

What are 3 other stores in your area?

Shopping: Problem solving

1. You are at the deli counter and want the ham that is on sale but are having trouble getting the right words out. What can you do?

2. You forgot you customer bonus card. The cashier asked for your phone number so she can look it up. You are having trouble saying your phone number correctly. What can you do?

3. You have a coupon for buy one get one free but when you checked out the discount didn't show up and you were charged full price. What would you say to the cashier?

4. You used the motorized cart to do your shopping but can't grab something up high. What could you ask somebody as they walk by?

5. You want to go to the store and shop on your own but your family is worried and wants to come with you. What could you tell them?

Shopping:

1. You have a 20% off coupon for one item at Bed Bath and Beyond. You want to buy a bathroom mat that costs $20. Once you use the coupon how much will the bath mat cost?

2. The grocery store offers online shopping with drive up pickup service for $4..99 each time. They also offer the service for a year with unlimited pickup for $99. If you use the online/pickup service at least once a week, which option is a better value?

3. You have $500 budgeted to spend on groceries every month. You go to the store 8 times each month. How much can you spend each visit if you divide the money equally?

4. You have $40 you can spend at Walmart. You want to buy sunglasses, a hat, suntan lotion, and water bottle. After you buy all the items on your list, how much money do you have left?
   - hat $5.99
   - sunglasses $11.99
   - sun tan lotion $8.99
   - water bottle $3.99

Money Management:

Monthly Budget:

Bill	Company	Amount
Phone		
Cell Phone		
Cable		
Power		
Gas		
Trash		
Internet		
Water		
Car payment		
Mortgage/Rent		
Car insurance		
Other:		
Other:		
Totals:		

Monthly Bills:

Bill	Carrier	Amount	Payment Method
Phone			
Cell Phone			
Cable			
Power			
Gas			
Trash			
Internet			
Water			
Car payment			
Mortgage/Rent			
Car insurance			
Other:			
Other:			
Totals:			

Monthly Budget:

Bill	Carrier Name	Phone Number	Address	Website/ Email
Phone				
Cell Phone				
Cable				
Internet				
Power				
Trash				
Water				
Mortgage/ Rent				
Car Payment				

Bill	Carrier Name	Phone Number	Address	Website/ email
Car Insurance				
Gas				
Other				
Other				
Other				
Other				
Other				
Other				
Other				
Other				

Online Bill Management:

Bill	Website	Log In	Password

Budget Planning Worksheet:

Bills		
Housing		
Mortgage/ Rent		
Second Mortgage		
Real Estate Taxes		
Repairs/Maintenance		
Homeowner/Renters Insurance		
Utilities		
Electricity		
Gas		
Water		
Trash		
Cell Phone		
Internet		
Cable		
Land Line		

Budget Planning Worksheet:

Food	Plan	Actual
Groceries		
Restaurants		
Clothing		
Self		
Family		
Car		
Car Payment		
Car Payment		
Gas		
Maintenance		
Car Insurance		
Personal		
Life Insurance		
Health Insurance		
Savings		
Entertainment		

Budget Planning:

1. Your Internet provider charges $20 a month for the first 6 months and $30 a month after that. You agreed to a two year contract when you signed up. How much will two years of Internet service cost?

2. Gas prices dropped from $3.60 a gallon to $1.99 a gallon over the last three months. How much cheaper is gas per gallon now?

3. You just purchased a new car that had a promotional interest rate of 0%. You financed $20,000 of the car's price and received a 5 year loan. What will your monthly car payments be?

4. You want to save $3000 to go on a family vacation. You are able to save $200 a month for the vacation. How long will it take to save enough money to go?

5. Amazon.com offers a subscribe and save service. A 48 pack of toilet tissue costs $24 for one time purchase. Subscribe and save service offers 5% off. What is the discounted price?

Budget: Practice phone calls

1. Call AT&T's customer service 1(800) 331-0500 and ask: "What does it cost to sign up for a shared value plan?"

2. Call 411 and get the phone number for you local power company or look it up on the internet.

3. Call Geico 1-800 793-2003 and ask how much it will cost for a pet insurance policy for two golden retrievers.

4. Call Direct TV at 1855-229-4388 and how much it costs for their best package.

5. Call your local Department store and ask their operating hours on Sunday.

6. Call a pizza place of your choice and ask what specials they are offering.

Budget: Banking

Check Number	Date	Transaction	Withdrawal	Deposit	Balance
		Balance Forward			

Add the following transactions to the check book register:

You Start the month with $1000 in your account.

January 1, 2016 you wrote check #144 for $900 to cover your rent.

January 3, 2016 you deposited $500 from Michael Smithson.

January 6, 2016 you wrote check #145 for $200 for your car payment.

January 10, 2016 you wrote check #146 for $100 to Duke Power.

January 15, 2016 you made a deposit of $1500 from your employer.

January 20, 2016 you wrote check #147 for $75 for the cable bill.

Budget: Banking

Check Number	Date	Transaction	Withdrawal	Deposit	Balance
		Balance Forward			

Add the following transactions to the check book register:

You start the month with $2000 in your account.

February 1, 2016 you wrote check #148 for $1100 to cover your rent.

February 3, 2016 you deposited your $2000 paycheck.

February 6, 2016 you wrote check #149 for $300 for your car payment.

February 10, 2016 you wrote check #150 for $100 to Piedmont Power.

February 15, 2016 you made a deposit of $2000 from your employer.

February 20, 2016 you wrote check #151 for $75 for the cable bill.

Budget: Banking

Check Number	Date	Transaction	Withdrawal	Deposit	Balance
		Balance Forward			

Add the following transactions to the check book register:

You start the month with $1500 in your account.

March 1st you wrote a check for $1000 to cover your rent.

March 3rd you deposited your $2500 paycheck.

March 6, you wrote check #170 for $200 for your car payment.

March 10, you wrote check #171 for $200 the Utilities Company.

March 15 you made a deposit of $2500 from your employer.

March 20 you wrote check #151 for $100 for the cable bill.

Restaurant Outings:

Order a meal from the following menu:

Brooke's BBQ

Appetizers

BROOKE'S SAMPLER PLATTER

St. Louis style spareribs are just the starter with fried chicken tenders, chili-roasted corn fritters, onion strings and traditional or boneless wings tossed in your choice of sauce.

CHICKEN TENDERS

Crisp, golden-brown chicken tenders tossed in Brooke's special seasoning and served with our own honey bbq sauce.

CHILI-ROASTED CORN FRITTERS

Classic southern favorite with jalapeno and chili roasted corn. Served with clover honey for the perfect sweet heat combination.

SMOKED SALMON SPREAD

Our own hickory-smoked salmon, cream cheese, capers and chipotle peppers makes this a spread worth swimming upstream for. served with fire grilled flatbread.

SOUTHSIDE RIB TIPS

A full pound of tips, hickory smoked and fire grilled served on a bed of our famous fries with a side of jalapeno pickled red onions, hell fire pickles and our southside bbq sauce.

ONION STRINGS

Lightly breaded and flash fried, served with New Orleans-style remoulade sauce.

SALADS

All entree salads served with a warm, freshly-baked corn bread muffin brushed with a honey-butter glaze.

BBQ SALAD

Your choice of barbeque pulled chicken, Texas beef brisket or Georgia chopped pork on a bed of crisp greens, smoked bacon, cheddar cheese, diced tomatoes and tossed with our house made honey bbq dressing.

CRISPY CHICKEN SALAD

Garden greens topped with fried chicken tenders, crisp bacon, grated cheddar, tomatoes and shoestring potatoes tossed with our house made honey bbq dressing.

GRILLED CHICKEN CAESAR SALAD

a chilled platter of crisp romaine lettuce tossed in our own Caesar dressing topped with sliced, grilled chicken breast.

SMOKED SALMON CAESAR SALAD

Dig into the ultimate caesar salad: featuring crisp romaine lettuce freshly tossed in Brooke's own caesar dressing and topped with chilled, hickory smoked salmon.

BBQ CHOPPED SALAD

iceberg and romaine tossed with cilantro, shredded cheddar, tomato, roasted corn, black beans, fried tortilla strips and our own lime chipotle ranch dressing then drizzled with rich & sassy. with hot grilled chicken breast.

SIDE SALAD

(fresh garden or caesar).

SANDWICHES

Our sandwiches are served with pickles and your choice of one side. For just $0.99 we ll top your sandwich with creamy coleslaw.

GEORGIA CHOPPED PORK SANDWICH

Our award winning, slow smoked chopped pork topped with rich & sassy bbq sauce.

BARBEQUE PULLED CHICKEN SANDWICH

Hand pulled chicken tossed in rich & sassy sauce and topped with melted jack cheese.

HICKORY CHICKEN SANDWICH

Marinated chicken breast, grilled and topped with jack cheese and two strips of smoked bacon.

CAJUN CHICKEN SANDWICH

Grilled chicken breast with pepper jack cheese, piled high with fried onion strings and topped with New Orleans style remoulade sauce.

CHAR GRILLED CHICKEN SANDWICH

Marinated chicken breast with crisp lettuce and tomato.

HOT LINK SAUSAGE

Smoked and spicy a mouthful of hollers on a bun.

TEXAS BEEF BRISKET SANDWICH

Piled high with hand-seasoned, hickory smoked Texas beef brisket.

SMOKED SIRLOIN TRI-TIP SANDWICH

Sliced hickory-smoked tri-tip served on a toasted hoagie roll with Texas pit horseradish sauce.

BURGERS

Our 1/2 pound burgers are seasoned 100% ground beef patties, grilled medium-well and served with pickles and your choice of one side. Substitute a turkey burger for any of our ground beef burgers.

ULTIMATE BBQ BURGER

A juicy ground beef patty beneath a pile of Georgia chopped pork with two strips of jalapeno bacon, melted sharp American cheese and our signature Beam & cola bbq sauce.

SPICEY BURGER

Careful, this cow kicks. A seasoned burger slathered with spicy bbq sauce and topped with melted pepper jack cheese, jalapeno bacon and hell fire pickles.

TRUE BLEU CHEESEBURGER

Bleu cheese lovers, meet the cheeseburger of your dreams. A flame-grilled patty on a toasted bun with lettuce, tomato, red onion and topped with both tangy bleu cheese dressing and crumbles.

TURKEY BURGER

A meaty burger that's really lean. Now you're talkin' turkey. Premium ground turkey on a toasted bun loaded with lettuce, tomato, red onion and our special bbq mayo.

BROOKE'S FAVORITE BURGER

Melted jack cheese, two strips of smoked bacon and Brooke's favorite sauce. Rich & sassy atop a char grilled burger.

CHAR GRILLED CHEESEBURGER

A classic burger, served with lettuce, tomato and your choice of melted jack or sharp American cheese.

Chicken Wings

TRADITIONAL WINGS

Brooke's traditional wings specially seasoned and tossed in your choice of sauce.

BROOKE'S AMAZINGLY BONELESS WINGS

No bones about it. These bbq wings are amazingly meaty all the way through. Tossed in your choice of sauce.

BBQ Classics

Served with corn bread and your choice of two sides.

GEORGIA CHOPPED PORK

Smoked for up to 12 hours and chopped to order, our award-winning bbq pork is juicier than a Georgia peach.

SOUTHSIDE RIB TIPS

Afull pound of tips, hickory smoked and fire grilled with a Memphis style dry rub. Served with a side of jalapeno pickled red onions, hell fire pickles and our southside bbq sauce.

BEER BATTERED COD

Beer battered and breaded with a special blend of cornmeal and panko breadcrumbs. Served with our house made spicy pickle tartar sauce.

CHICKEN TENDERS

Crisp, golden-brown chicken tenders tossed in Brooke's special seasoning and served with our own honey bbq sauce.

HOT LINK SAUSAGE

A real mouthful of hollers. Twelve ounces of hot link sausage best served with an ice cold beer to douse the flames.

Feasts

ALL AMERICAN BBQ FEAST

A full slab of St. Louis-style spareribs, a whole country-roasted chicken, 1/2 lb. of either Texas beef brisket or Georgia chopped pork, creamy coleslaw, famous fries, wilbur beans, four corn-on-the-cob and four corn bread muffins. Served family-style for 4-6.

FEAST FOR TWO

All the flavor, but half the size of our All American BBQ Feast. Served family-style for 2-3.

Bar B Que

Hand-rubbed with Brooke's secret blend of tongue-tingling special spices and pit-smoked for 5-6 hours over a smoldering hickory fire.

THE BIG SLAB

Served with corn bread muffin and your choice of two sides. (the big slab 12 bones, 1/2 slab 6 bones, 1/3 slab 4 bones).

BABY BACK RIBS

Slow smoked, seasoned with our Chicago style rib rub, then sauced with sweet & zesty. One bite of these babies, and you've got a mouthful of hollers.

BIG BABY

Served with corn bread muffin and your choice of two sides. (1/2 slab).

Sauces

RICH & SASSY

Brooke's original sauce with a blend of hand-picked herbs and spices. Heat level - mild.

BUFFALO

Our traditional buffalo-style sauce with a nice flavorful kick. Heat level - medium.

DEVIL'S SPIT

a devilishly good hot sauce loaded with chili peppers and spices. heat level - medium high.

PINEAPPLE RAGE

grilled pineapple blended in a sauce with habanero peppers. Hot, sweet and dangerously delicious. heat level - medium high.

Side Dishes

BAKED BEANS

Baked beans loaded with smoked pork, brisket, hot link sausage and jalapeno peppers.

CREAMY COLESLAW

A zesty slaw that's pineapple sweet with a hint of horseradish.

GARLIC RED SKIN MASHED POTATOES

Red skin potatoes mixed with milk, butter and garlic.

POTATO SALAD

Potatoes with red onion, celery, hard cooked egg, mayonnaise and a hint of mustard.

CORN ON THE COB

Buttery, super sweet cobettes.

Desserts

BREAD PUDDING

Melt in your mouth, scratch-made bread pudding and pecan praline sauce served warm with vanilla bean ice cream.

HOT FUDGE KAHLUA BROWNIE

Warm, walnut covered chocolate brownie soaked with Kahlua liqueur and topped with vanilla bean ice cream, hot fudge and whipped cream.

SWEET DIXIE MINIS

Save room for one of Brooke's after dinner minis. Choose famous bread pudding, Kahlua brownie or strawberry shortcake, each served with vanilla bean ice cream and whipped cream.

BETTER THAN MOMS PECAN PIE

Sticky, rich Georgia pecan pie, served warm with vanilla bean ice cream and whipped cream.

FAMOUS SUNDAE

Vanilla bean ice cream drizzled with hot fudge or pecan praline sauce and topped with whipped cream.

DRINKS

Coke, Diet Coke, Sprite, Diet Sprite, Mug Root Beer, Sweet Tea, Unsweet Tea, Cherry Coke,

BBQ Menu Questions:

1. Order an appetizer, salad, side and desert.

2. What main dish could you order that can feed 6 people?

3. How big are the burgers?

4. If you don't like red meat, what options do you have if you want a burger?

5. Which mini desert would you like?

6. Which BBQ sauce is mild? Which one is the spiciest?

7. How long do they cook their BBQ?

8. What also comes with the BBQ Classics?

BBQ Menu Questions:

9. What two sides would you pick?

10. How many different chicken sandwiches do they offer?

11. What salad should somebody with a seafood allergy avoid?

12. What diet sodas are on the menu?

13. You want to order for your table of four. What will you order? One of your friends is a vegetarian.

14. Your check comes to $44. You would like to tip 15%. How much is the tip? How much is the total?

15. If the bill comes to $35 and you want to tip 20% how much is the tip?

Avery's Italian Place

Subs

HAM, AMERICAN CHEESE $5.99

BUFFALO CHICKEN $6.79

HAM, CAPPACOLA, SALAMI, PROVOLONE $6.59

VEGGIE - TOMATO, MUSHROOM, ONION, PEPPERS, PROVOLONE $6.29

HAM, SALAMI, TURKEY, PROVOLONE $7.79

TURKEY, PROVOLONE $7.19

CHICKEN CLUB $6.69

Hot Subs

CHICKEN PARMESAN $6.69

MEATBALL PARMESAN $6.69

SAUSAGE PARMESAN $6.69

EGGPLANT PARMESAN $6.69

VEAL PARMESAN $7.59

STEAK & CHEESE $7.49

add peppers, mushrooms or onions 30c ea.

PIZZA SUB (MOZZARELLA CHEESE, PIZZA SAUCE) $5.99

additional toppings. 30c ea.

Children's Menu 12 and under

SPAGHETTI WITH MEATBALLS $4.49

ZITI WITH TOMATO SAUCE $3.99

SPAGHETTI WITH BUTTER $3.99

PIZZA SLICE & GARLIC KNOT $2.60

FINGERS & FRIES COMBO $5.49

Bottle Beer

DOMESTIC $2.99
IMPORTED $3.49

Beverages

REGULAR $1.99
CHILDREN'S CUP $1.79
IBC ROOT BEER $1.99
CAN SODA $1.29
2 LITER SODA $2.49
APPLE JUICE $1.29

Desserts

CANNOLI $3.59
fresh homemade - chocolate or vanilla
CHEESECAKE $3.99
TIRAMISU $3.99
ALMOND CREAM CAKE $3.99
PECAN CARROT CAKE $3.99
CHOCOLATE ESPRESSO CAKE $3.99
CHOCOLATE TRUFFLE CAKE $3.99
CHOCOLATE CHIP COOKIE $1.49

Pizza

Toppings offered: pepperoni, sausage, black olive, eggplant, green peppers, banana peppers, fresh mozzarella, bacon, onion, ham, spinach, broccoli, chicken, tomato, mushroom, meatball, ground beef, jalapeno, pineapple, garlic, fresh basil.

14" MEDIUM (CHEESE) $11.09

16" LARGE (CHEESE) $3.15

SICILIAN (CHEESE) 14" SQUARE $14.60

ADDITIONAL TOPPINGS EA. $1.50

EXTRA CHEESE $2.00

BY THE SLICE $2.50

additional toppings 35c ea.

Specialty Pizza

no substitutions

MEAT LOVERS$17.09 - $19.15

pepperoni, sausage, ground beef and ham

SPINACH, TOMATO & GARLIC$15.59 - $17.65

VEGGIE LOVERS$17.09 - $19.15

mushroom, green pepper, tomato & onion

HAWAIIAN$17.09 - $19.15

pineapple, ham, black olive & cheddar

WHITE$14.09 - $16.15

mozzarella and ricotta, garlic & oil

PIZZA MARGHERITA $15.59 - $17.65

roma tomatoes, fresh mozzarella, fresh basil, olive oil

BUFFALO CHICKEN $17.09 - $19.15

diced chicken w/wing sauce, mozzarella cheese. Blue cheese or ranch dressing on the side

BBQ CHICKEN $17.09 - $19.15

diced chicken w/BBQ sauce, red onions and cheddar cheese

Appetizers

MUSSELS FRA DIAVLO $6.99
FRENCH FRIES $2.79
CHICKEN FINGERS$5.79 - $7.49
MOZZARELLA STICKS $5.79 - $7.49
FINGERS & FRIES COMBO $7.29
BACON & CHEESE FRIES$5.29 - $2.00
HOT SEAFOOD ANTIPASTO $9.99
mussels, calimari, shrimp and scallops

Antipasto & Salads

dressings: ranch, blue cheese, French, honey mustard, 1000 Island, Italian & fat free ranch. Additional dressing .50 each

TOSSED SALAD $3.79
CHEF SALAD $8.59
GRILLED CHICKEN SALAD $6.79
CAESAR SALAD $4.79
LARGE ANTIPASTO $9.99
SMALL ANTIPASTO $6.99
ADD CHICKEN TO ANY SALAD $3.00

Chicken Wings

mild, hot or BBQ. Extra celery & dressing .50 each.
SINGLE (10) $6.49
DOUBLE (20) $12.98
TRIPLE (30) $18.99
GRAND SLAM (50) $29.99

Garlic Knots & Bread

GARLIC KNOTS $3.50
GARLIC BREAD $7.99

Pasta

includes salad and garlic knots. Substitute caesar salad at no cost or Greek salad at $2.00 additional cost.

LASAGNA $10.99
MANICOTTI $10.49
RAVIOLI $10.49
BAKED ZITI $9.99
BAKED ZITI SORENTINA (RICOTTA) $10.99
BAKED ZITI SICILIAN (EGGPLANT) $10.99
SPAGHETTI WITH WHITE OR RED CLAM SAUCE $10.99
SPAGHETTI OR ZITI WITH TOMATO SAUCE $8.99
SPAGHETTI PARMESAN $9.99
SPAGHETTI OR ZITI $9.99
with one of the following -meat sauce, meatballs, sausage, or mushrooms
SPINACH MANICOTTI $9.99
LOBSTER RAVIOLI $13.99
served in vodka sauce
TORTELLINI ALFREDO $9.99
PENNE ALA VODKA $11.99

Chicken Entrees

includes salad & garlic knots

MARSALA $13.49
Chicken breast sauteed in marsala wine, garlic and shallots, smothered with fresh chopped mushrooms, served over spaghetti
SCALLOPINI $13.49
Chicken cutlet sauteed in garlic and shallots with a lemon butter sauce, smothered with sliced mushrooms, served over spaghetti
FRANCESE $13.49
Boneless breast of chicken battered and sauteed in a lemon butter sauce, served over spaghetti

CACCIATORE $13.49

Boneless breast of chicken sauteed in marinara sauce with green peppers, mushrooms and onions, served over spaghetti

PICCATA $13.49

Chicken cutlet sauteed in a lemon butter sauce with garlic, shallots and capers, served over spaghetti

PARMESAN $13.99

boneless breast of chicken lightly breaded, smothered with homemade tomato sauce and mozzarella cheese, served with a side of spaghetti

Seafood Entrees

includes salad & garlic knots

SHRIMP OR CALAMARI MARINARA $13.99

Shrimp or calamari sauteed in Avery's homemade marinara sauce, served over spaghetti

MUSSELS MARINARA $12.99

Mussels sauteed in marinara sauce, served over spaghetti

SHRIMP ALFREDO $13.99

Shrimp served in a creamy alfredo sauce, served over spaghetti

SHRIMP SCAMPI $13.99

A generous serving of jumbo shrimp, sauteed in lemon butter with shallots, garlic, and a touch of red pepper, served over spaghetti

SHRIMP PARMESAN$13.99

A generous serving of shrimp, smothered with a homemade tomato sauce and mozzarella cheese, served with a side of spaghetti

SEAFOOD MEDLEY $14.99

Shrimp, calamari, scallops sauteed in marinara, shallots, garlic with a touch of crushed pepper (spicy!). Served over spaghetti

Restaurant Outings:

Avery's Italian Restaurant Menu Questions:

1. Does this restaurant serve beer?
2. What two types of sub sandwiches do they serve?
3. What brand of root beer do they serve?
4. Is there a children's menu?
5. What comes with the Seafood Entrees?
6. How many different types of seafood are in the Seafood Medley? Name them.
7. How many inches is a large pizza?
8. What shape is the Sicilian Pizza?
9. How much does an order of garlic knots cost?

10. What is the total cost if you order a Caesar salad, lasagna, domestic bottle of beer and cheesecake?

Item	Price
Total:	

10. How much will it cost if add a Greek Salad to a Pasta Entree?

11. Does it cost any extra to add a Caesar salad to a Pasta Entree?

12. How much does it cost to add chicken to a salad?

13. Describe the chicken marsala dish.

14. The waitress comes to the table and says, "Can I start you off with anything?" What would you say?

15. You finished your meal. Your waitress asks if you would like anything else. What would you say?

16. You ordered the Lobster Ravioli. It is overcooked and tastes like it has gone bad. What would you say to your waitress?

17. Place a dessert order for you and two friends.

18. How much is a large pizza with 4 extra toppings?

19. If you order an appetizer, drink, entree of your choice what would the total cost be plus a 15% tip?

Entree	Price
Total	
Total + Tip	

Schedules: Activity Schedule

Time	Monday	Tuesday	Wednesday	Thursday	Friday
9 am	tea social	bridge	group walk	shopping	tea social
10 am	trivia	exercise	knitting	exercise	trivia
11 am	crafts	singer	manicures	bridge	poker
12 pm	lunch	lunch	lunch	lunch	lunch
1 pm	book club	shopping	trivia	raffle	gardening
2 pm	rummikub	trivia	video game	aerobics	crochet
3 pm	chess	darts	pool table	bridge	music
4 pm	art class	bingo	yoga	bingo	walk
5 pm	dinner	dinner	dinner	dinner	dinner
6 pm	movie	poker	chess	movie	darts
7 pm	pokeno	movie	happy hour	bible study	star gazing

1. What activity is available Thursday at 2pm?

2. When are the two shopping outings?

3. You like card games. What and when are your choices?

4. You want to do something outdoors. What and when are your choices?

5. When can you get a manicure?

6. What happens at Tuesday at 11 am.

7. When is the book club meeting?

8. A friend wants you to join her for bingo. You don't want to play. What could you tell her?

9. What time do the activities start everyday?

10. When is the last activity?

11. How many times a week is there a happy hour?

12. How many times a week do they have bingo?

13. Would you rather go to knitting or art class?

14. You have a Dr. appointment on Thursday at 2pm. What activities will you miss if it takes you 30 minutes to get there?

15. What nights do they show movies? Is the movie always at the same time?

16. What days and times is trivia?

17. What happens at Friday at 7 pm? Would you like to go?

18. If you went on the shopping trip, where would you like to go?

19. What time do they have chess?

20. What kinds of exercise classes are available?

Senior Center Activity Schedule

Activity Location Key: AU Auditorium, CO Conference Room, FR Fitness Room, LO Lobby, CA Card Room, C1 Craft Room1, GA Gallery, PA Patio, CL Computer La,b C2 Craft Room2, GM Game Room

Time	Monday	Tuesday	Wednesday	Thursday	Friday	Saturday
8	Quilter's Club C2	Dominoes CA	Chorus Practice AU	Bingo CA	Bingo CA	Woodcarving CI
9	Knit/ Crochet CA	Dominoes CA	Morning Tea CA	Bingo CA	Line Dance AU	Dance Class FR $5
10	Knit/Crochet	Dominoes CA	Chair Exercise AU	Bingo CA	Chair Exercise AU	Dance Class FR
11	Depart for Art Musuem Rembrant exhibit	Chair Exercises AU	Bridge AU	Chorus Practice AU	Adaptive Yoga LO Mats Provided	Computer Class C2
12	Line Dance AU	Bible Study CO	Poker CI	Movie AU	Symphony AU	Lunch outing to Cracker Barrel
1	Clay Class C2	Bridge GM	Rummykub GM	Valentine's Day Crafts C1	Ice Cream Social AU	Square Dance AU

Activity Management:

1. How much does the line dance cost?

2. Do you need to bring your own mats to yoga class?

3. Where is the clay class held

4. What activity is on Tuesday at 10 am?

5. What is the exhibit at the art museum outing on Monday at 11 AM?

6. What time do the activities start?

7. What time are the last activities of the day?

8. What day of the week is the Senior Center closed?

9. What is available on Thursday at 11 am?

10. Are all the activities free?

11. If you could attend three activities, what would they be?

12. Where and when is the lunch outing?

13. What group game activities are available?

14. What exercise opportunities are there?

15. What arts and crafts activities are on the schedule?

16. What month is the schedule for? How do you know?

17. Where is the symphony performance located?

18. When and where is the computer class?

19. How long does Bingo last on Thursday?

20. What day is there morning tea?

Class Registration: Practice filling out the registration form for an activity of your choice:

Participant Name: _____ If Under 18-Age: ____ School: _____

Class Barcode Number or Name: Time: Day: Cost: Location Code

1._____   _____ _____ $_____   _____

2._____   _____ _____ $_____   _____

3._____   _____ _____ $_____   _____

4._____   _____ _____ $_____   _____

Name: _____ Parent or Guardian: _____

Address: _____ City/State:_____ Zip: _____

Home Number: _____ Work Number: _____

Emergency Contact Name: _____ Emergency Contact Number: _____

Email Address: _____ Second Phone Number (optional): _____

Class Name	Time	Day	Cost	Location Code
Water Aerobics	8 AM	Monday	$5	P1
Water Aerobics	8AM	Friday	$5	P1
Water Aerobics	10 AM	Thursdays	$5	P1
Salsa Class	1pm	Monday	$5	S1
Tango Class	3pm	Tuesdays	$5	S2
Square Dancing	5pm	Tuesday/Thursday	Free	S1
Quilting Club	11 Am	Wednesday	Free	CR1
Crochet Corner	9 am	Tuesday	Free	CR2
Yoga	10 am	Monday/Wednesdays	$5	S3
Wine Tasting	5 pm	Fridays	$10	CR1

Maps:

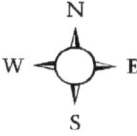

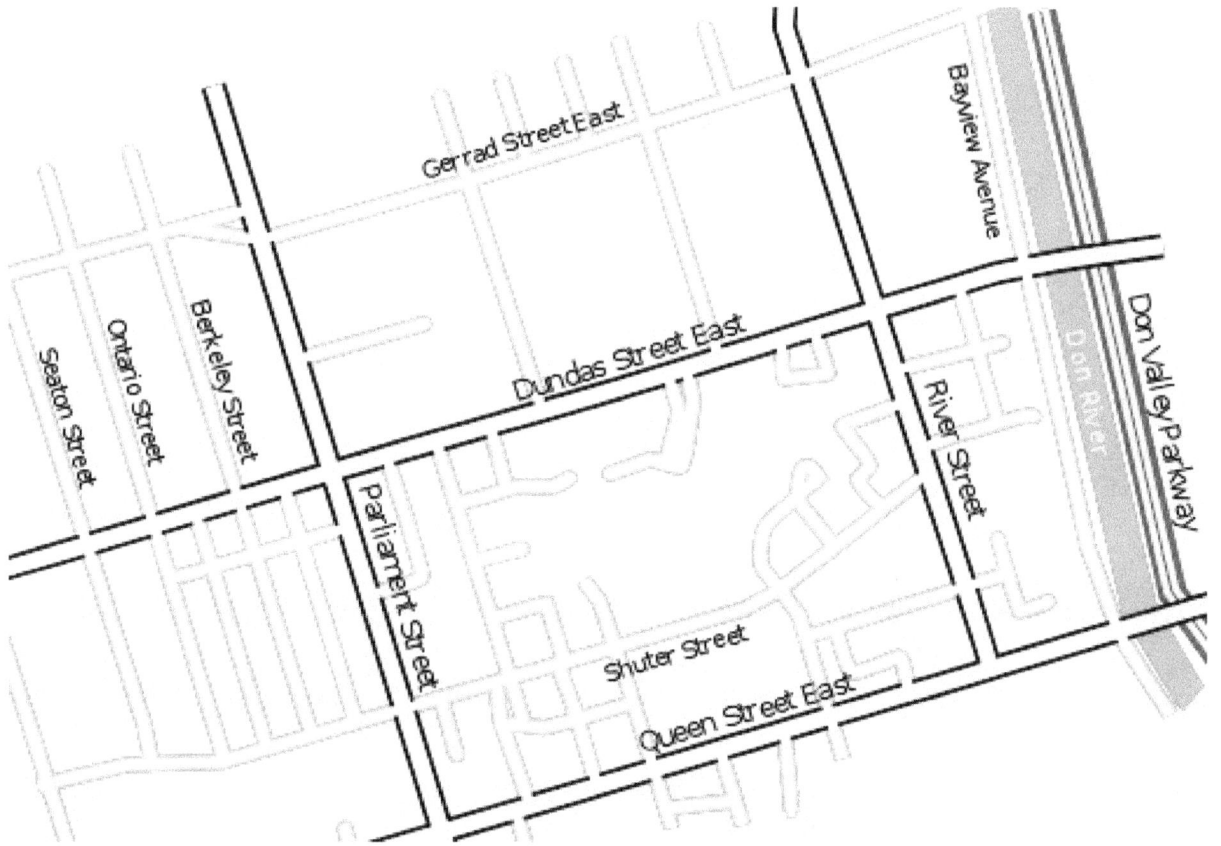

1. What street lines the Don River on the East Side?

2. What street is between Seaton Street and Berkeley Street?

3. If you follow Dundas Street East towards the river and take a right onto River Street, what street is the second one on your right?

4. Name 4 streets that travel east to west.

5. Name 7 streets that travel north to south.

Maps:

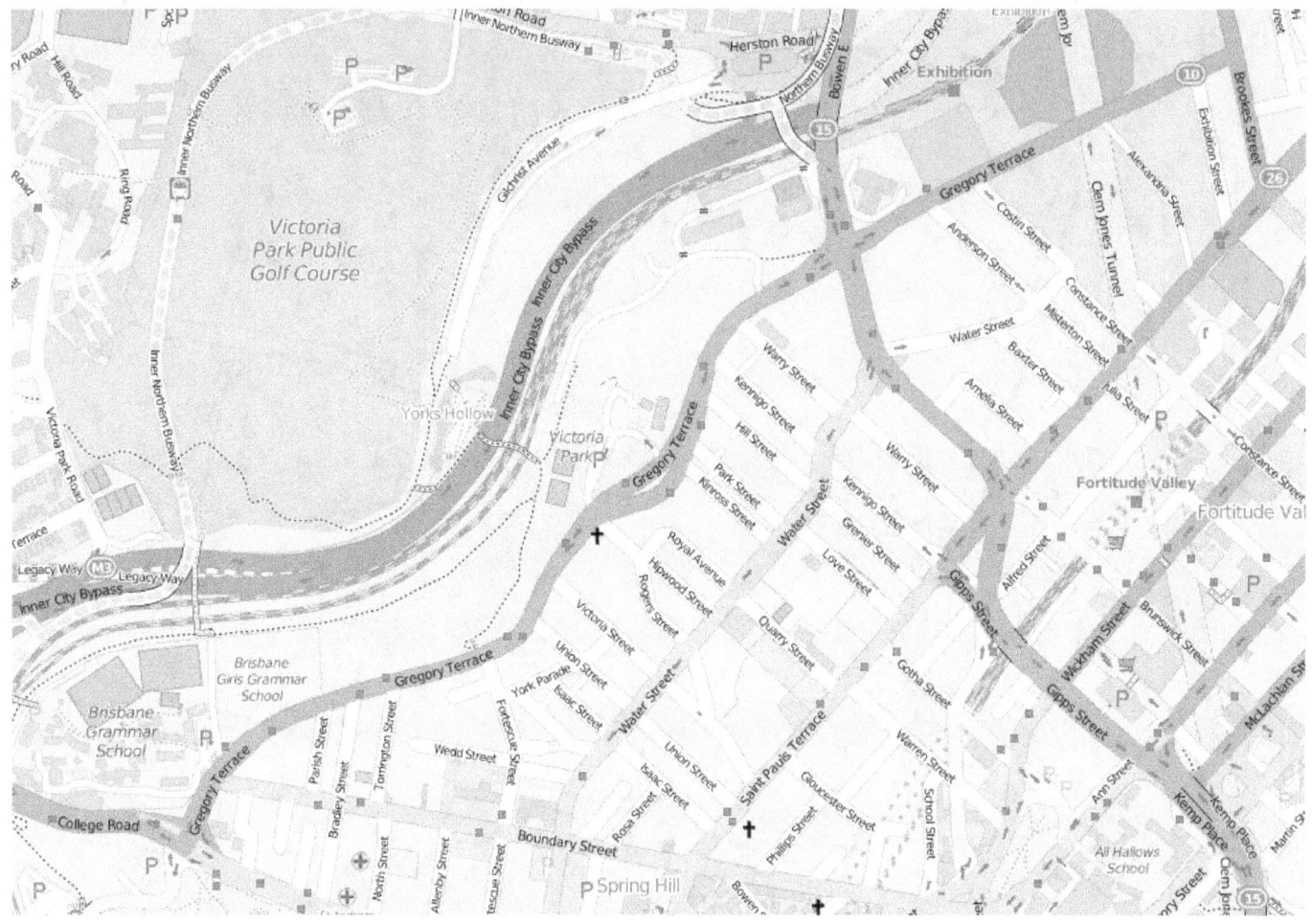

1. What is the name of the public golf course?

2. What bus route runs through the park?

3. How many parking lots are in Victoria Park?

4. Is the school south of the park for boys or girls?

5. How many bridges cross over the Inner city Bypass?

6. Draw a line north on Gregory Terrace, turn right onto Hill Street, left onto Water Street, and then right onto Constance street. What is the name of the tunnel that Constance Street crosses over?

7. How many shopping centers are on the map?

Maps:

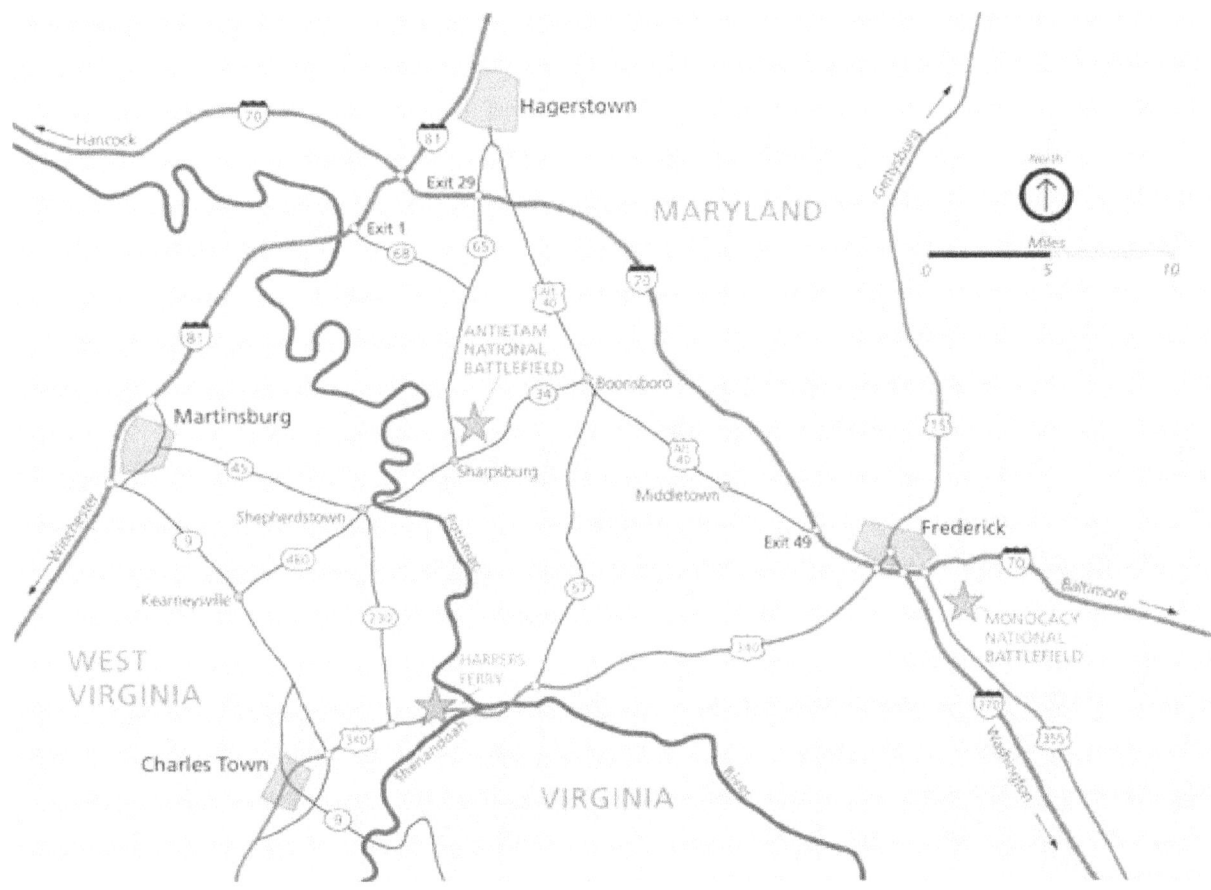

1. About how many miles long is the portion of highway 81 on this map?

2. What two highways run through Frederick Maryland?

3. Where do the Potomac River and Shenandoah River meet?

4. How many States are on this map?

5. What historic site is furthest south on the map?

6. Which battlefield is further East?

7. What road is off exit 1 from highway 81?

8. You want to visit Harper's Ferry. What road would you need to take?

Maps:

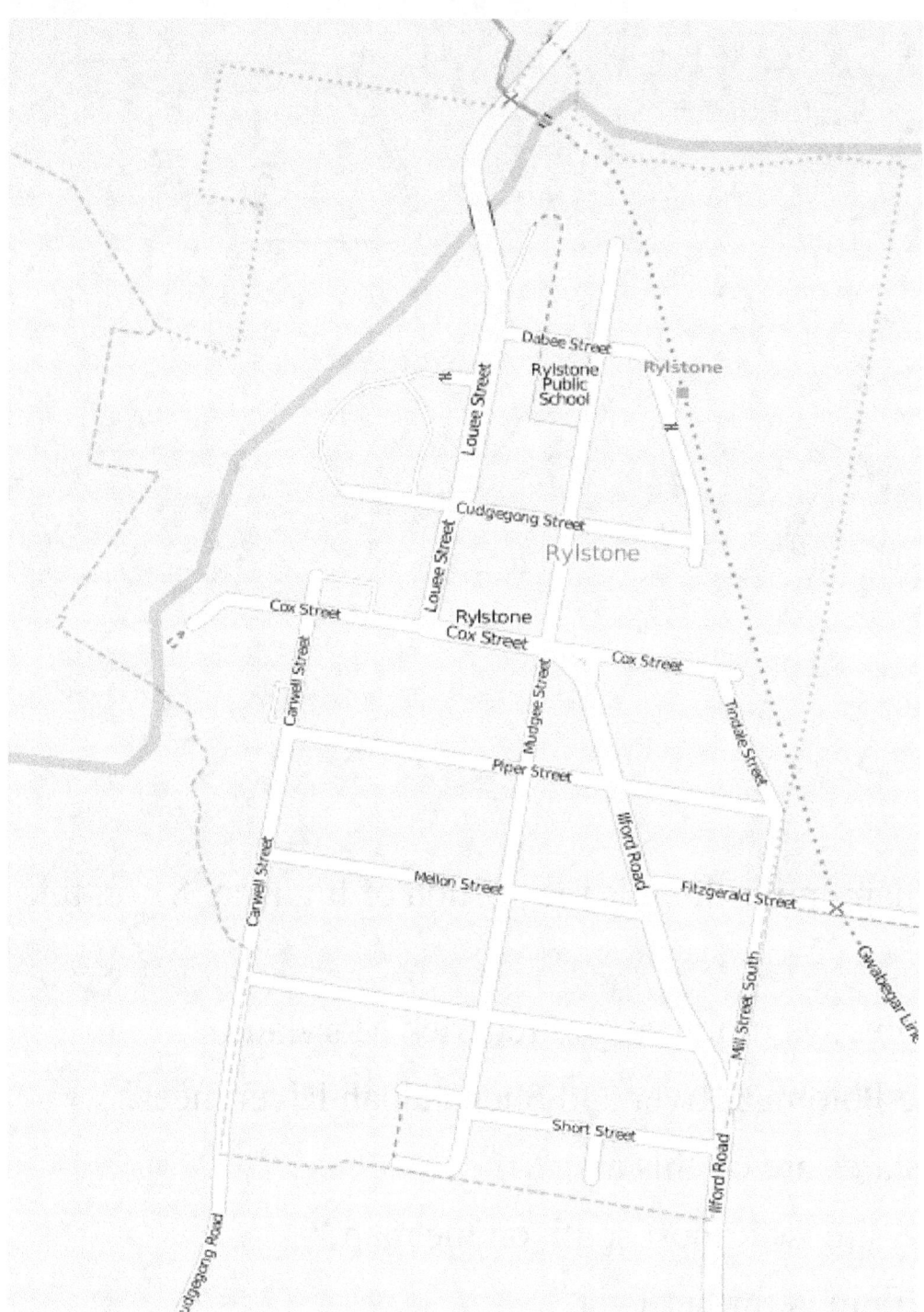

1. Draw an X at the intersection of Mudge St and Piper St.

2. Circle the school.

3. How many streets intersect with Mudge Street?

Maps:

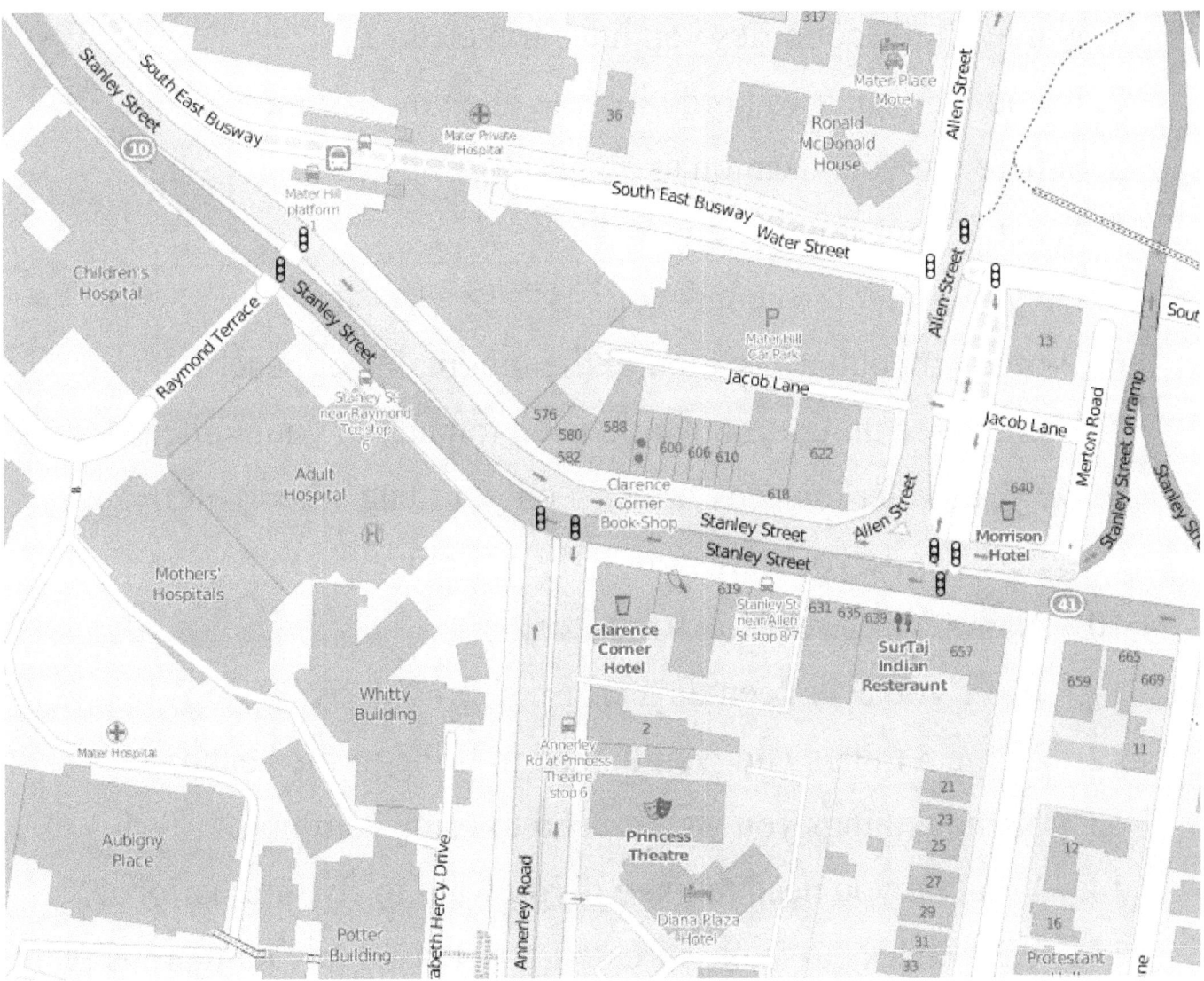

16

1. Draw a path from the Princess Theatre to the Ronald McDonald House.

2. How many buildings are in the hospital complex?

3. How many bus stops are on the map?

4. Draw a line from the Children's Hospital to the Morrison Hotel?

16 http://commons.wikimedia.org/wiki/File:Open_Street_Map_-_Clarence_Corner.JPG

Travel:

1. Name all the countries you have traveled to.
2. Name the countries bordering the one you live in.
3. Where did you vacation as a child?
4. What is your favorite city?
5. Do you prefer the country or city?
6. Would you rather vacation in the mountains or beach?
7. Name three things you would need to pack in your suitcase.
8. Do you prefer to check or carry on your bag when you fly?
9. Where would you rather go, Italy or France? Why?
10. Name 3 different ways to travel.
11. Have you ever been on a cruise ship?
12. Name 5 things you would need to bring to the beach.
13. Name 5 things you would need to bring camping.
14. What do you need to have if you want to fly international?
15. Who checks to make sure you don't bring any dangerous plants or animals into a country?
16. Describe the process of going through security.
17. Name a famous National Park in the United States.
18. What is a popular place to visit in New York City?
19. How would you book a vacation online?
20. Name 3 rental car companies.

Travel:

Name the famous place (convergent naming)

1. An group of islands in the pacific ocean that is a 50th State in the USA. The island is home to indigenous Polynesian people with a rich culture and history known for luaus, the hula dance and beautiful flower leis. The islands have amazing beaches, mountains and waterfalls. During World War II, the Japanese bombed Pearl Harbor.

2. This is a popular travel destination in China. It is the only man made structure that can be seen from space. Construction began in 200 BC and the structure is over 5,000 miles long. It runs along the northern border of China.

3. This is one of the 7 wonders of the world. It is a palace in India that sits next to the Yamuna River. It is a large white building with a dome on the top and is actually a mausoleum. You can see the building's reflection in the pool in front of it.

4. This is a National Park in South Dakota with the faces of 4 American Presidents carved into the rock of the mountainside.

5. This is a popular vacation site in Nevada. It is famous for a strip of hotels with gambling and elaborate entertainment shows. It is known for the slogan "What happens is _____ stays in _____."

6. This is a city in France. It is know for the Eiffel Tower, Louvre, Champs-Elysees and the Nortre-Dame Cathedral.

7. This is a giant waterfall between Ontario and New York State. It is the most powerful waterfall in North America.

8. This is a popular beach destination in Mexico. It is on the coast of the Yucatan Peninsula. College students from the US, flock here for spring break vacations.

9. This city is in Washington State. It is typically very raining there. It is a seaport city and know for Starbucks coffee and the Space Needle.

10. This is a city in Italy. It is known as a "floating city." It is known for gondolas, artwork and unique beauty.

11. This is a place where you take children. You will find amusement rides here with many characters including princesses. The entrance is a castle and it is called "the most magical place on earth." You would see many images of Mickey Mouse here.

12. This is an island off of San Francisco Bay near the Golden Gate Bridge. It used to be a prison. It is sometimes referred to as "The Rock."

13. This is a place that everyone can enjoy. Many cities and towns have them. You could see a giraffe or and elephant here. Children love to visit them and see animals from all over the world.

14. This is a famous part of New York City. You would go here to see a play like Les Miserables or Rent.

Bus Schedule:

	Bus Schedule Spring 2014			
	MONDAY, TUESDAY, WEDNESDAY AND THURSDAY			
TRIP	DEPART MAIN CAMPUS FOR GEORGE	ARRIVE GEORGE	DEPART GEORGE TO MAIN CAMPUS	ARRIVE MAIN CAMPUS
1	7:35 A.M.	7:50 A.M.	8:15 A.M.	8:30 A.M.
2	9:00 A.M.	9:15 A.M.	9:35 A.M.	9:50 A.M.
3	10:25 A.M.	10:40 A.M.	11:10 A.M.	11:25 A.M.
4	11:45 A.M.	12:00 P.M.	12:10 P.M.	12:25 P.M.
5	12:40 P.M.	12:55 P.M.	1:10 P.M.	1:25 P.M.
6	2:00 P.M.	2:15 P.M.	2:35 P.M.	2:50 P.M.
7	3:25 P.M.	3:40 P.M.	4:00 P.M.	4:15 P.M.
8	5:30 P.M.	5:45 P.M.	6:05 P.M.	6:20 P.M.
9	6:50 P.M.	7:05 P.M.	7:25 P.M.	7:40 P.M.
10	8:20 P.M.	8:35 P.M.	8:55 P.M.	9:10 P.M.

1. You want to arrive at George at 11am. What time do you need to leave the main campus?

2. You need to arrive at the main campus by 3pm. What time do you need to depart George?

3. You have a meeting at the main campus at 5pm. It takes you 20 minutes to walk from the bus stop to the location of your meeting. What time do you need to depart from George to get to your meeting on time?

4. How long does it take to get from George to the Main Campus?

5. Does the bus run on Fridays?

Charlotte International Airport Departure Schedule

Destination	Flight	Airline	Departure Time	Terminal	Status
HSV Huntsville	US5283	US Air	9 AM	E14A	On Time
PHL Philadelphia	AA664	American Airlines	9:07 AM	C6	Delayed
AUS Austin	US5537	US Air	9:10 AM	E26	On Time
ORD Chicago	AC8600	Air Canada	9:15 AM	A11	On Time
SAV Savannah	US5154	US Air	9:18 AM	E3	Delayed
SAV Savannah	AA567	American Airlines	9:20 AM	C10	on Time
JFK New York	AB37	Air Berlin	9:22 AM	E4	On Time
JFK NEW York	US7345	US Air	9:25	E25	Delayed
JFK New York	AA1830	American Airlines	9:27	C14	Cancelled

1. How many flights go to New York City?

2. Which one is cancelled?

3. How many different airlines are on this schedule?

4. What is the flight status of the flight to Austin?

5. Your Ticket says flight AB37. Where are you going and what Terminal do you need to go to?

6. What time does the flight to Chicago leave?

TSA Liquid Rule

You are allowed to bring one small bag of liquids, aerosols, gels, creams and pastes through the checkpoint. These are limited to 3.4 ounces or less per container. Consolidating these containers in the small bag separate from your carry-on baggage enables TSA officers to screen them quickly.

3-1-1 for carry-ons. Liquids, gels, aerosols, creams and pastes must be 3.4 ounces (100ml) or less per container; must be in 1 quart-sized, clear, plastic, zip-top bag; 1 bag per passenger placed in screening bin. The bag limits the total liquid volume each traveler can bring.

Declare larger liquids. Medications, baby formula/food and breast milk are allowed in reasonable quantities exceeding three ounces, and they don't have to be in the zip-top bag. Declare these items for inspection at the checkpoint. TSA officers may need to open them for additional screening.

If in doubt, put your liquids, gels, aerosols, creams and pastes in checked baggage.

Inbound international flights

You may now carry liquids more than 100 mL in your carry-on bag if:

- You are traveling internationally into the United States with a connecting flight;
- they are in transparent containers;
- you bought them at a duty-free shop, and
- the store packed them in a secure, tamper-evident bag.If your liquids are not in a secure, tamper-evident bag, you must pack them in your checked bag. If the liquids alarm during screening, we will need to screen them further.

1. You want to bring a bottle of shampoo on your carry on bag. How many ounces does it have to be.

2. Can you bring liquids more than 100 ml if you are coming to the U.S. on an international flight and it is in a transparent container?

3. Can you bring liquid medication that is larger than 3 ounces?

4. How many ml are in 3.4 ounces?

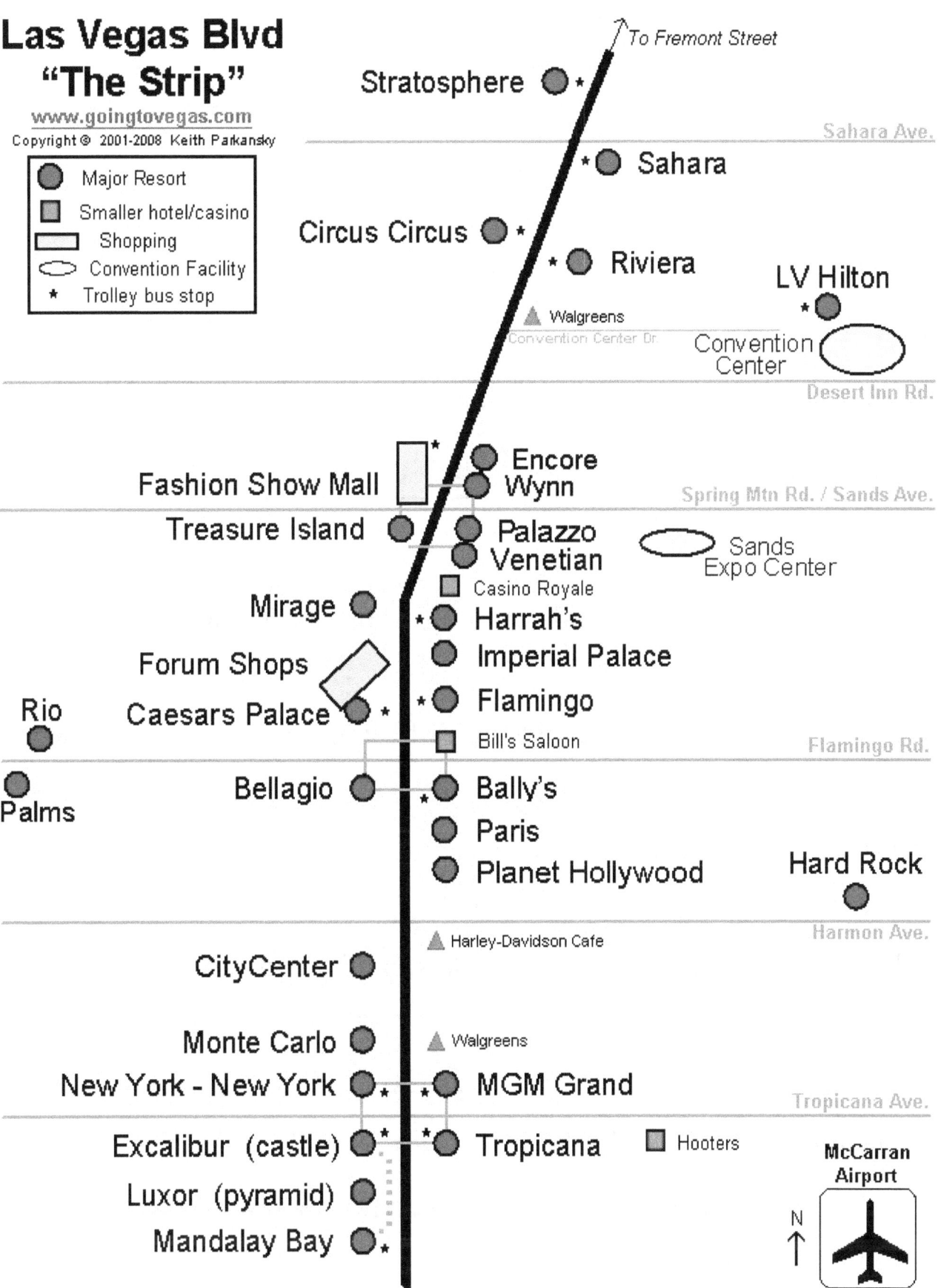

Las Vegas Blvd
"The Strip"

www.goingtovegas.com
Copyright © 2001-2008 Keith Parkansky

●	Major Resort
■	Smaller hotel/casino
▭	Shopping
⬭	Convention Facility
★	Trolley bus stop

To Fremont Street

Stratosphere ● ★

Sahara Ave.

★● Sahara

Circus Circus ● ★

★● Riviera

LV Hilton
★●

Walgreens
Convention Center Dr.

Convention Center

Desert Inn Rd.

Fashion Show Mall ★
● Encore
● Wynn

Spring Mtn Rd. / Sands Ave.

Treasure Island ● ● Palazzo
● Venetian

Sands Expo Center

■ Casino Royale

Mirage ●

★● Harrah's

Forum Shops

● Imperial Palace

Caesars Palace ● ★ ★● Flamingo

Rio ●

■ Bill's Saloon

Flamingo Rd.

Palms ●

Bellagio ● ★● Bally's

● Paris

● Planet Hollywood

Hard Rock ●

Harmon Ave.

Harley-Davidson Cafe

CityCenter ●

Monte Carlo ● Walgreens

New York - New York ● ★ ★● MGM Grand

Tropicana Ave.

Excalibur (castle) ● ★ ★● Tropicana

Hooters ■

McCarran Airport

Luxor (pyramid) ●

N ↑

Mandalay Bay ● ★

Hotel Booking: Use the map for reference.

Hotel	Price per night.
Bally's	$149
Planet Hollywood Hotel	$239
Harrah's	$75
Mandalay Bay	$199
Bellagio	$240

1. You have a budget $1000 for 5 nights at a hotel. Which above hotels fit your budget?

2. You want to stay at a hotel South of Flamingo Rd. What are your choices?

3. What hotel is the least expensive?

4. What hotel is the most expensive?

5. How much would you save if you stayed at Harrah's for 5 nights instead of Mandalay Bay?

6. You want to be close to the Sands Expo Center for a convention. What hotel on the list is closest to the Expo?

7. In addition to price, what other considerations would you keep in mind when booking a hotel?

Communication Practice:

1. Call Enterprise Rent a Car: 1-800-264-6350 and ask, "How much will it cost to rent a compact car from JFK airport in New York for 5 days."

2. Call the Four Seasons Hotel in Washington DC and ask if they have any available rooms for this coming Friday and Saturday night. Phone:1-202-342-0444

3. Call the Seattle Airport 1-800-544-1964 and ask what assistance they provide for somebody in a wheelchair.

4. Call the San Francisco Zoo 1-415- 753-7080 and find out what there hours are on a Sunday.

5. Call Carnival Cruise Line 1 -888- 227-6482 and find out what port is closest to you.

Computer Travel Practice:

1. Go to Expedia.com and find out how much it would cost to stay at the Sheraton Waikiki, on Waikiki Beach, HI for five nights a month from now.

2. Use tripadvisor.com to read a review of the restaurant Bouley in New York, NY.

3. Use Orbitz.com to book a flight to Miami and a hotel on South Beach in Miami for 5 nights.

4. Use google.com to find out what are the 7 wonders of the world. Write them here:

_____   _____

_____   _____

_____   _____

_____

Delta Wheelchair Services

We can accommodate a variety of types of chairs to ensure that you feel secure at every point in your journey.

Airport Wheelchairs

Delta has wheelchairs available for use at airport locations; request this service when making reservations. Upon arrival at the airport, simply notify a Delta representative that you require a wheelchair for transportation to the departure gate.

Aisle Chairs

Specially-designed aisle wheelchairs make it easy for our non-ambulatory passengers to reach their seat when boarding and deplaning our aircraft. If you think you need this service, please request it when making reservations so we can have the aisle chair available at your departure gate.

Onboard Wheelchairs

Every one of our mainline aircraft includes an onboard wheelchair specially designed to fit the aisle of the aircraft and for use to and from the lavatory. Flight attendants are trained in the operation of this wheelchair and will assist you with its use. (They are not, however, required to lift or carry you.) This onboard wheelchair is not used outside the aircraft; if you need a wheelchair at a connecting point, arrangements can be made in advance via Reservations.

Alternative Boarding Devices

Stairways are sometimes used for boarding instead of loading bridges. If you are unable to ascend or descend steps, let a Delta representative know, and we will provide an alternative boarding method.

Delta Electric Cart Service

Electric carts are available at some major airports, including Atlanta, Cincinnati and New York (JFK Airport). These carts are available for use by semi-ambulatory passengers who have difficulty walking long distances; carts can pick-up and drop-off passengers throughout the terminal or concourses.

Travel Accommodations:

1. What airline are the services provided by?
2. What will Delta provide if you are unable to use the stairway to the airplane?
3. In what cities are electric cart services available?
4. If you need a wheelchair to get to and from the airplane lavatory, what service is available?
5. Will the airline attendants help you get in and out of the wheelchair?
6. You don't usually use a wheelchair but you are worried you will be unable to walk the distance of the airport to and from your gate. What services are available?
7. What will you need to do if you need a wheelchair when you arrive at your destination?
8. What is special about the on-board wheelchair?
9. Can you bring an over-sized wheelchair onto the plane?
10.   Will you be able to sit in the emergency exit aisle?

Travel and Packing:

Make a list of things you would need for a trip to your relatives house.

_____

_____

_____

_____

_____

_____

_____

_____

_____

_____

_____

_____

_____

Travel and Packing: Make a list of things you would bring on a family vacation to the beach. You are driving so don't forget big items.

_____

_____

_____

_____

_____

_____

_____

_____

_____

_____

_____

_____

_____

_____

Travel and Packing:

Put the appropriate letters next to the correct item for each trip. Use more than one symbol when appropriate.

Beach- B   Ski Trip-S   Camping- C

Suntan Lotion:_____

Canteen:_____

Sun Glasses:_____

Gloves:_____

Snow Boots:_____

Hiking Boots:_____

Boogie Board:_____

Lounge Chair:_____

Sun Hat:_____

Bug Spray:_____

Toilet Paper:_____

Winter Coat:_____

Matches:_____

Tent:_____

Flip Flops:_____

Bathing Suit:_____

Wool Socks:_____

Backpack_____

Travel Descriptions:

Define each of the items on the list.

Suitcase	Passport
Fanny Pack	Traveler's Checks
Dramamine	Carr-on Bag
Security Scan	Duty Free Shop
Tray Table	Oxygen Mask
Subway	Taxi
GPS	Concierge
Bellboy	Compass
Travel Insurance	Valet
Flight Attendant	Amenity
Pilot	Overhead Compartment
Bed and Breakfast	Embassy
Frequent Flier	Terminal
Itinerary	Late Check Out
Nonstop	Room Service
House Keeping	Suite
Tourist	Standby

Travel Itinerary: Destination: Cancun Mexico

Departing Flight

Date	Time	Airline	Confirmation #	Departure	Gate	Arrival Time	Arrival City
5/15	8:05 AM	Southwest	HD228Q	Baltimore BWI	C2	10:50 AM	Dallas DFW
5/15	11:40 AM	Southwest	SW6745	Dallas DFW	D7	4:10 PM	Cancun Mexico

Hotel Shuttle

Date	Time	Company	Confirmation #	Pick Up Location	Destination	Duration
5/15	4:30	Super Shuttle	B7789	Baggage Claim	Fiesta Americana Coral Beach	20 minutes

Hotel Information

Date	Check in time	Confirmation #	Hotel	Address	Room	Check Out
5/15	5:00 PM	Z77821	Fiesta American Cancun Coral Beach	Boulevard Kukulkan Km 9.5, Zona Hotelera, 77500 Cancún,	C301	5/22 11 AM

Returning Flight

Date	Time	Airline	Confirmation #	Departure	Gate	Arrival Time	Arrival City
5/22	1:20 PM	Southwest	HR4457	Cancun	A1	4:15PM	Dallas DFW
5/22	5:00 PM	Southwest	SW27845	Dallas DFW	C5	9:10 PM	Baltimore MD BWI

Answer the questions using the itinerary:

1. What city will you leave from?

2. What time will you need to arrive at the airport?

3. How many stops does your flight have?

4. Where are you going?

5. How long are you staying?

6. What airline are you traveling with?

7. What city does your connecting flight land in?

8. What gate is your connecting flight leaving from?

9. Your connecting flight arrives in Dallas at gate D1. Will you have to travel far to get to your departing gate for your flight to Cancun?

10. How will you get from the Cancun Airport to your hotel?

11. Where will you meet your shuttle driver?

12. What is the name of your hotel?

13. What is your room number?

14. Will you have to wait before you can check in to your room?

15. Cancun is in the Central Time Zone which is one hour earlier than Eastern Time in Baltimore. How long did your total flight time take?

16. What time will you leave the hotel to get to the airport for your returning flight?

17. You haven't booked your transportation to the airport for your returning flight. What are some of your options?

Itinerary

You are traveling from Chicago to San Francisco on US Air on March 15th. . Your flight Confirmation # is T5678. You leave at 9:30 from gate B7. The flight is 5 hours long. Your hotel shuttle is from the San Francisco Hilton and will meet you at baggage claim at 1 pm Pacific Time. You are staying 5 nights at the Hilton in room B109. Check-in is 3 pm. and check out is at 11 am. Your returning flight leaves at 8 AM from Gate B6 with US Air Confirmation # T57223. The flight is 5 hours long. Fill out your itinerary.

Departing Flight

Date	Time	Airline	Confirmation #	Departure	Gate	Arrival Time	Arrival City
						1	

Hotel Shuttle

Date	Time	Company	Confirmation #	Pick Up Location	Destination	Duration

Hotel Information

Date	Check in time	Confirmation #	Hotel	Address	Room	Check Out

Returning Flight

Date	Time	Airline	Confirmation #	Departure	Gate	Arrival Time	Arrival City

Home Management:

When you go on vacation. List several things you need to do to make sure your home is safe and in order.

_____   _____

_____   _____

_____   _____

_____   _____

List 8 different types of repair services for your home.

_____   _____

_____   _____

_____   _____

_____   _____

Make a list for your home insurance company of valuable items in your home.

_____   _____

_____   _____

_____   _____

_____   _____

Home Management: Carrier Phrases:

1. After dinner, I wash the _____.

2. In the fall the leaves clog up the rain _____.

3. The faucet sprung a leak. I need to call a _____.

4. I wanted more TV channels, so I ordered _____.

5. The carpet is getting dirty. I need to _____.

6. After I get up in the morning, I make the _____.

7. Every Thursday, I need to take the trash to the _____.

8. When it snows, I need to shovel the _____.

Home Management:

Describe how you would complete the following tasks.

Change a light bulb.

Change your vehicle's oil

Unload the dishwasher

Make spaghetti

Pay your phone bill

Mail a letter

Buy a new washer and dryer

Clean the windows

Mop the floor

Mow the lawn

Plant a garden

Organize a party

Get rid of termites

Decorate for the holidays

Do a delicate load of laundry

Clean the bathroom

Home Management: Computer Practice Tasks:

Find out how much it costs a month for cable and intranet from two different companies:

Company Name	Price

Using realtor.com, find the price of 3 homes for sale in your zip code.

House Address			
Price:			

Find a recipe to make a peach cobbler. Write the ingredients:

_____   _____   _____

_____   _____   _____

_____   _____   _____

_____   _____   _____

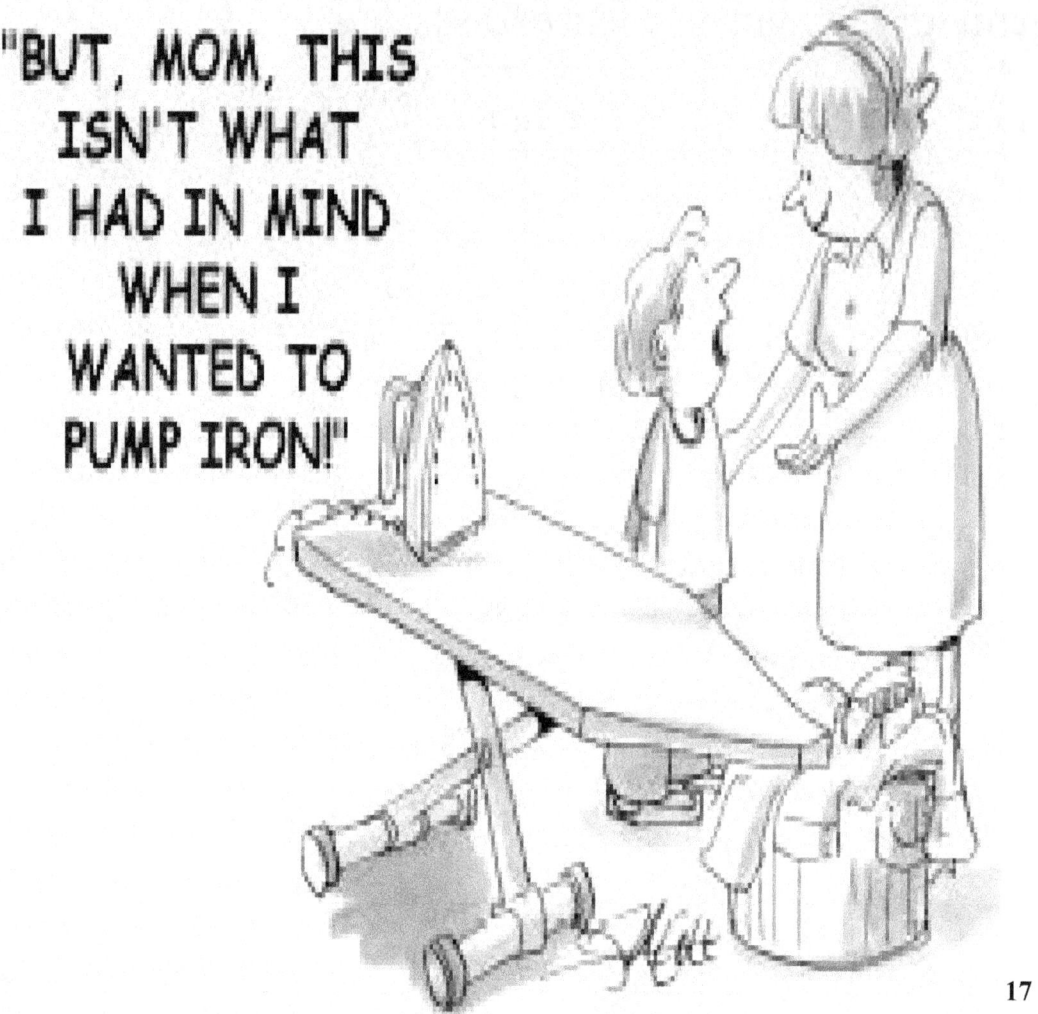

"BUT, MOM, THIS ISN'T WHAT I HAD IN MIND WHEN I WANTED TO PUMP IRON!"

1. What did the boy want to do?

2. What did his Mother have him do instead?

3. Describe how to iron a shirt.

Home Management:

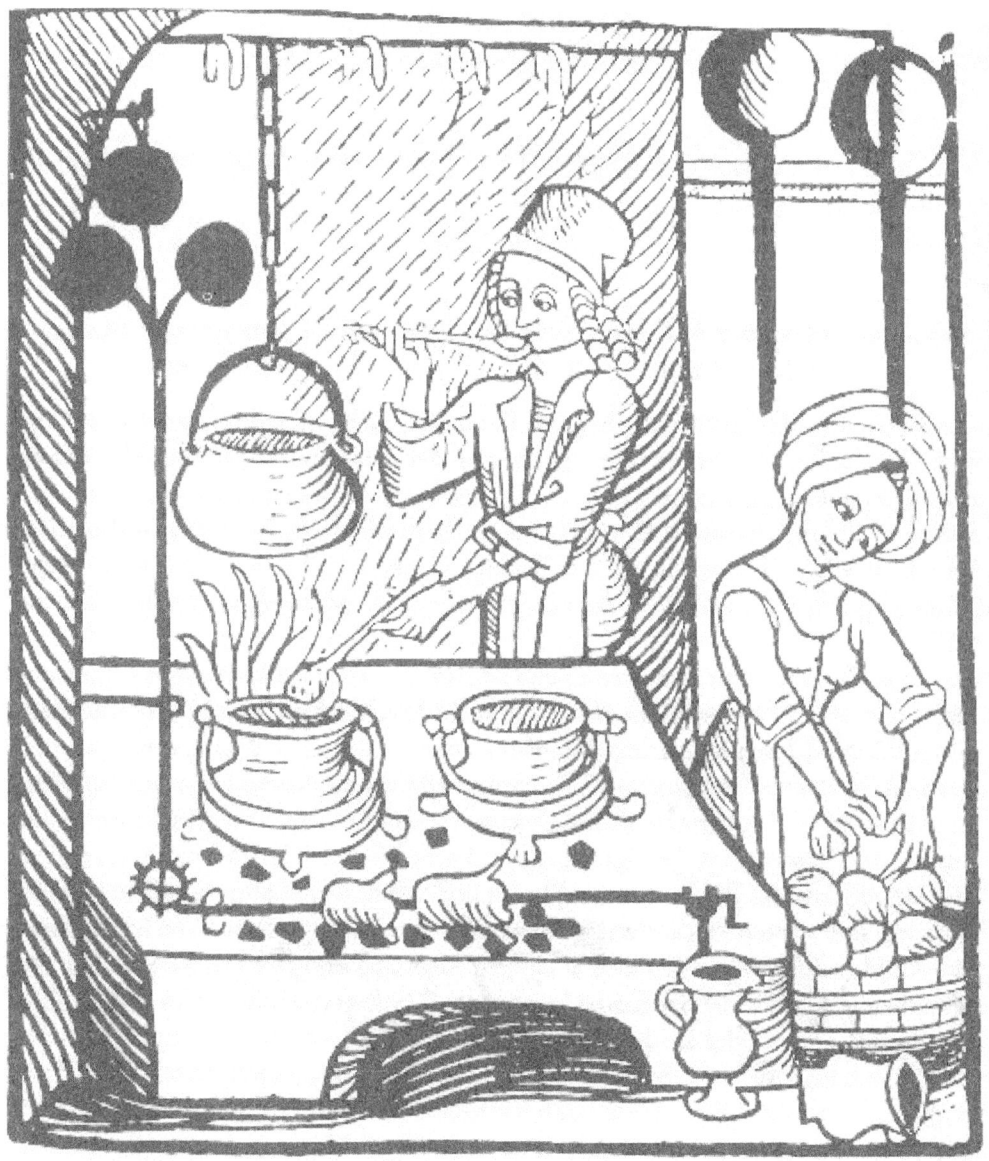

18

1. Describe what these women are doing.

2. Explain what is different about their kitchen from yours.

3. Name 5 different things in this picture.

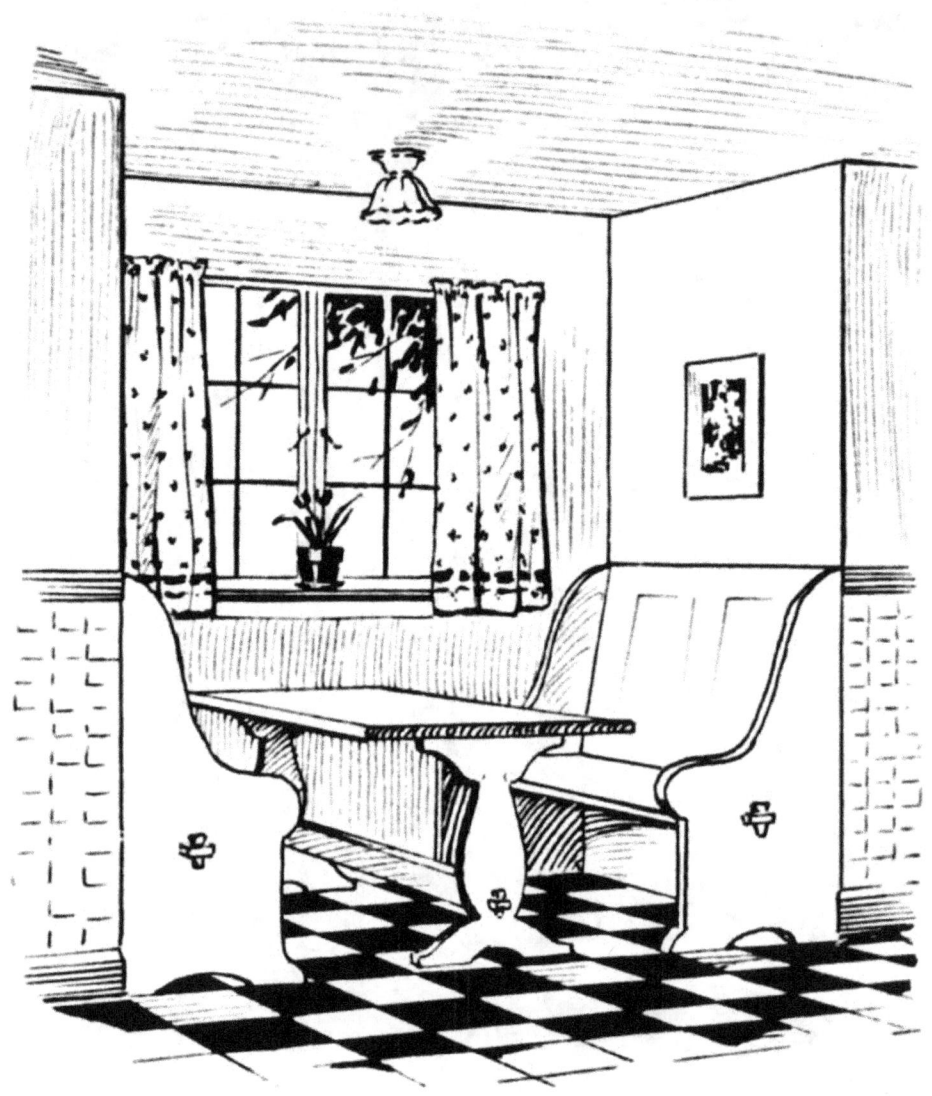

1. Describe the illustration.

2. How does this compare to your kitchen table?

3. Where might you find a table like this?

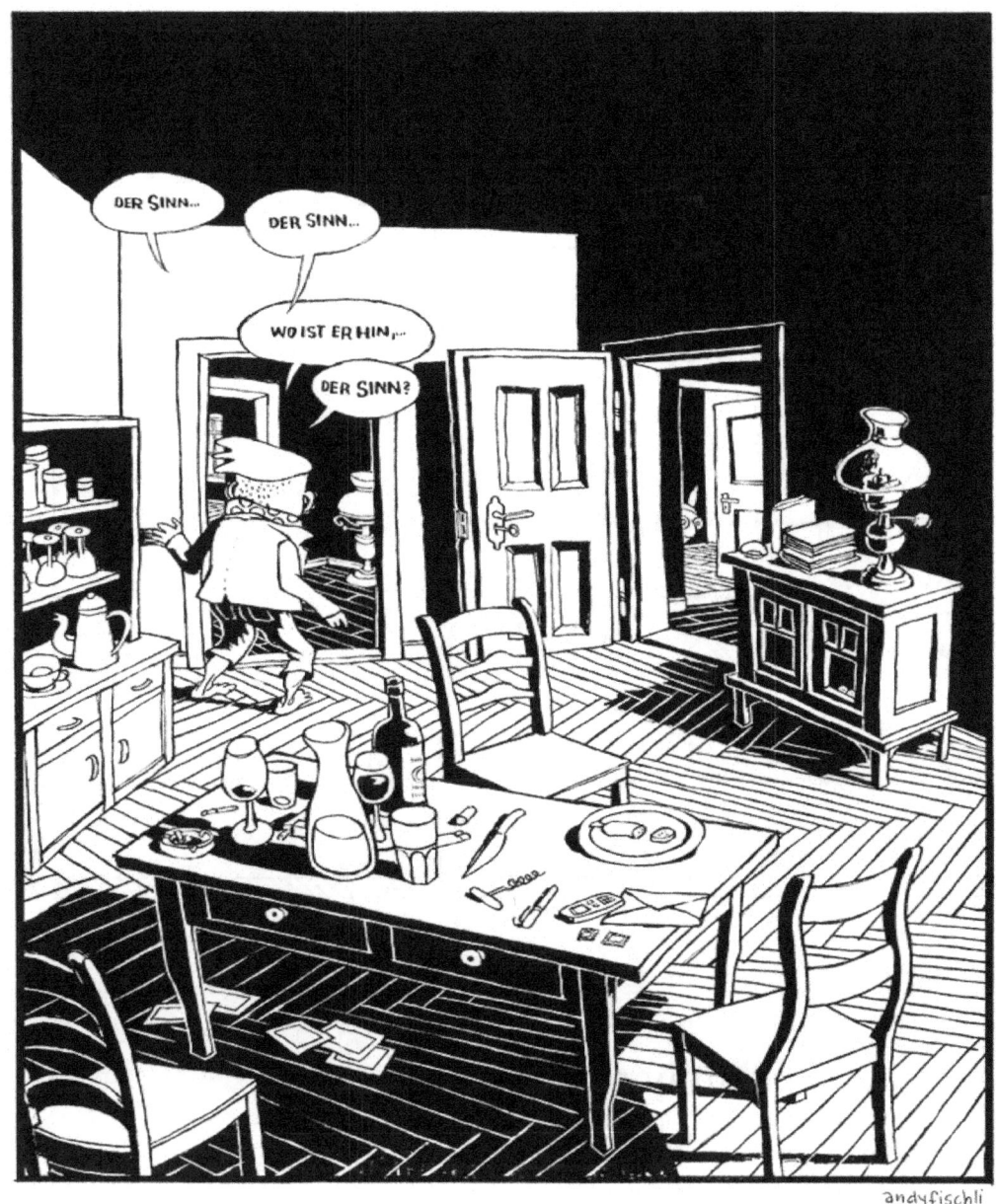

1. What do you think he is saying?

2. What was he doing at the table:

3. Name 10 items in the illustration.

4. Describe the room.

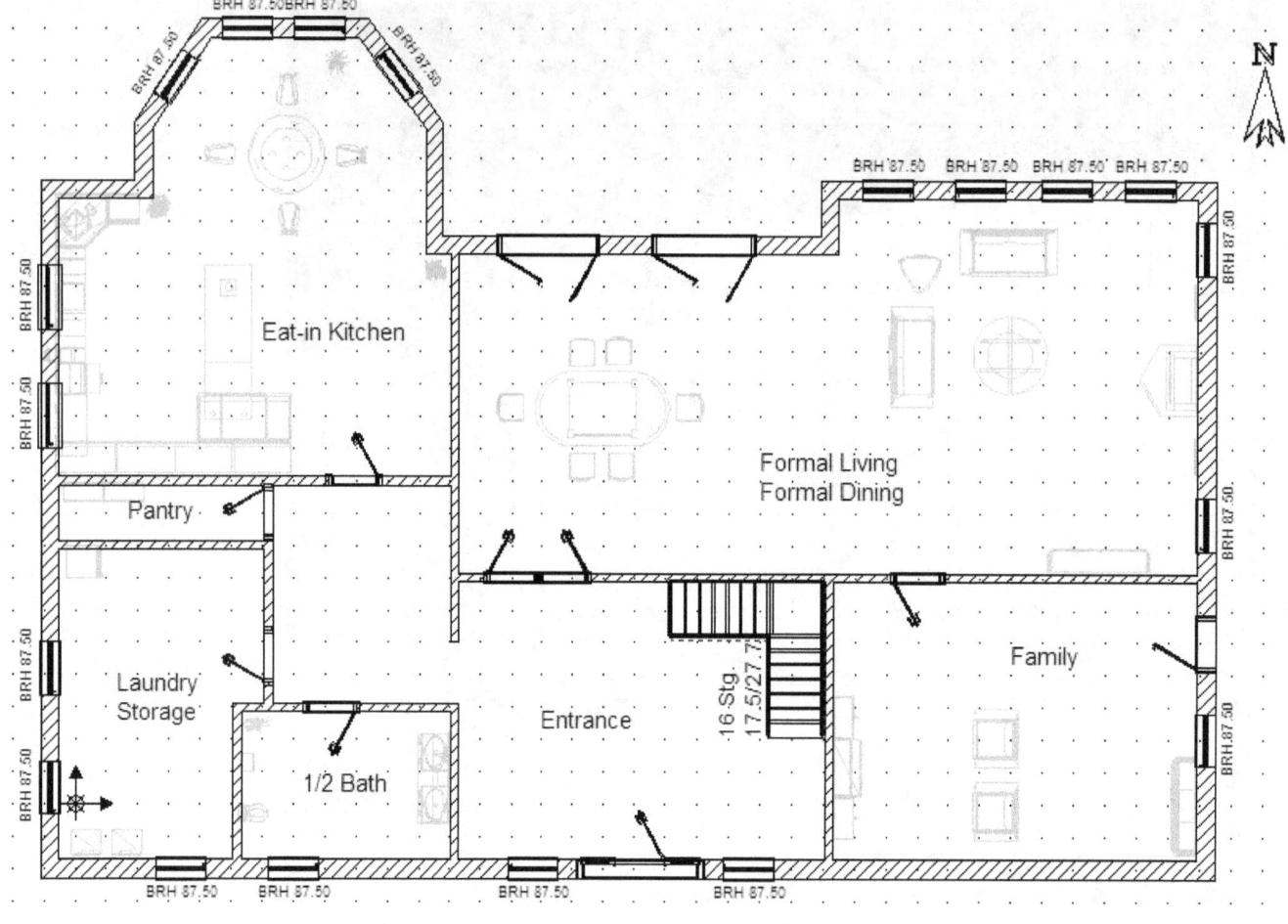

21

1. What furniture is in the family room?

2. How many windows are on this level?

3. What rooms connect to the kitchen?

4. Can you take a bath downstairs?

5. Are there any bedrooms on this level?

6. Put an X on the two tables.

7. Name 10 things you would put in the pantry.

8. Name two places where you would put a TV on this level?

21 Source:Boereck, CC-BY:http://commons.wikimedia.org/wiki/File:Sample_Floorplan.jpg

Sequence each task in the correct order:

Dishes

_____ Scrape the leftovers off the plates

_____ Put the dishes in the dishwasher

_____ Rinse the dishes in the sink

_____ Start the dishwasher

_____ Add the soap to the dishwasher

_____ Close the dishwasher door

Walk the Dog

_____ Open the door

_____ Put the leash and collar on your dog

_____ Clean up after your dog

_____ Bring a plastic bag

_____ Close your door

_____ Walk down the street

_____ Return home

Sequence each task in the correct order:

Brush Teeth:

_____ Put lid back on toothpaste

_____ Put toothpaste away

_____ Wet toothbrush

_____ Squeeze dime size amount of toothpaste on brush

_____ Rinse toothbrush

_____ Brush teeth

_____ Rinse out mouth with water

Put on Shoes and Socks

_____ Tie shoes

_____ Put on shoes

_____ Find socks

_____ Put socks on

Wash Your Hands

_____ Dry your hands

_____ Turn on the faucet

_____ Put soap on your hands

_____ Check temperature of water

_____ Lather up the soap

_____ Run your hands under the faucet for at least 20 seconds

_____ Turn on the faucet

Sequence: in the correct order:

Going to the Movies

_____ Pick out your seats

_____ Buy your tickets

_____ Select the movie you want to see

_____ Buy concessions

_____ Watch the movie

Write an email

_____ Log out

_____ Log in with your user name and password

_____ Write the email

_____ Select new email

_____ Type in the email address

_____ Press send

Laundry:

_____ Pour in the detergent

_____ Open the washing machine door

_____ Put the clothes in the washing machine

_____ Separate the the clothes

_____ Pour in the fabric softener

_____ Start the dryer

_____ Open the dryer door

_____ Close the washing machine door

_____ Take the wet clean clothes and put them in the dryer

_____ Start the washing machine

_____ Close the dryer

_____ Take out the clean dry clothes and put them away

Safety: Fall Prevention and Problem Solving:

Explain how to make each situation safer.

1. When you walk through your living space you have to walk around furniture.
2. You have several throw rugs on your floors.
3. Typically the floor has some papers and mail scattered around from your dog.
4. There are wires and cords on the floor where you walk.
5. Members of your family leave shoes and clothing on the steps with the intention of taking them upstairs later.
6. Your stairway is dark and is missing a light.
7. The top step is uneven.
8. Your stair handrail is loose.
9. Sometimes you slip a bit on the tub floor because it is slippery.
10. You need something to lean on or grab to get in and out of the tub.
11. The light near your bed is hard to reach.
12. The path from your bed to the bathroom is unlit.

If any of the items on the list apply to you, it is essential that you get help to fix the problem. These factors can increase your risk of falling and causing significant health and safety problems. Enlist the help of family members, home health aids and physical therapists to improve your safety and prevent falls. [22]

---

[22] Source: CDC from: http://www.cdc.gov/ncipc/pub-res/toolkit/checklistforsafety.htm

Safety: Fall Prevention

Explain how you can complete these recommendations from the Center for Disease Control to reduce your risk of falls:

-Exercise regularly. Exercise makes you stronger and improves your balance and coordination.

-Have your doctor or pharmacist look at all the medicines you take, even over-the-counter medicines. Some medicines can make you sleepy or dizzy.

-Have your vision checked at least once a year by an eye doctor. Poor vision can increase your risk of falling.

-Get up slowly after you sit or lie down.

-Wear shoes inside and outside the house. Avoid slippers.

-Improve the lighting in your home. Put in brighter light bulbs. Florescent bulbs are bright and cost less to use.

-It's safest to have uniform lighting in a room. Add lighting to dark areas. Hang lightweight curtains or shades to reduce glare.

-Paint a contrasting color on the top edge of all steps so you can see the stairs better. For example, use a light color paint on dark wood.

-Keep emergency numbers in large print near each phone. Put a phone near the floor in case you fall and can't get up.Think about wearing an alarm device that will bring help in case you fall and can't get up.

Safety: Swallowing

1. What are some strategies you can use to increase swallow safety?
   a. Take large sips
   b. Clear your throat between sips. Tuck your chin when you swallow
   c. Look up when you drink
   d. b and c

2. You notice you cough when you drink. Today you feel feverish. What should you do?
   a. Nothing, it is just a cold
   b. Tell your Doctor and have them scan your lungs
   c. Take some allergy medication
   d. Ask your doctor about getting speech therapy since you have had this problem for a long time.
   e. b and d

3. When you left the hospital, you were told to drink thick liquids. When you drink you should:
   a. Thicken all liquids with thickener powder
   b. Make sure not to swallow any water when you brush your teeth
   c. Order some pre-thickened juices
   d. Take your medication with thickened liquids
   e. All of the above

4. You had aspiration pneumonia. Aspiration pneumonia is:
   a. Just like regular pneumonia caused by germs in the air.
   b. Caused by food and or liquid getting in the lungs.
   c. Is very minor.

Safety: Swallowing

5. Some foods that can be dangerous if you have dysphagia are:
   a. popcorn
   b. steak
   c. lettuce
   d. hot dogs
   e. sausage
   f. all of the above

6. Thickened liquids are helpful because:
   a. They travel slowly giving you time to swallow.
   b. They are less likely to fall into the airway.
   c. They help prevent aspiration pneumonia.
   d. All of the above.

7. Dysphagia is:
   a. problems swallowing liquids
   b. problems swallowing solids
   c. difficulty chewing
   d. food pocketing in your mouth
   e. all of the above

8. If the Doctor and Speech Therapist recommend you need thick liquids, that means you should drink them:
   a. all the time
   b. only with meals
   c. only at night
   d. in everything except coffee

Life Participation:
Follow the steps to join a support group on Facebook for aphasia. Part of recovery involves pushing yourself to make new connections and prevent isolation. Aphasia Recovery Connection is a fantastic nonprofit organization that offers multiple resources to help with aphasia.

Step 1: Create an email account (If you already have email go to Step 2)

1. go to gmail.com
2. click create an account
3. Fill out the required fields to choose a user name and password. Make sure to write your user name and password down.

Step 2: Create a facebook account (If you already have a facebook account go to Step 3).
1. go to facebook.com
2. Click on the green sign up button.
3. Fill Out your information using your new email address
4. Click Sign Up
5. The first page will give you the option of finding friends. You can click on skip this step on the bottom right.
6. The next step gives you the option of uploading a photo for your facebook profile. You can also click on skip

Step 3: Join Aphasia Recovery Connection
7. In the white box next to the magnifying glass image write "Aphasia Recovery Connection". Click on the image below with the people's faces. This is the group page.
8. On the Aphasia Recovery Connection page, click on the white box on the upper right side that says "join group".

Life Participation:

You can also join the Facebook group:

Speech Therapy Aphasia Rehabilitation Group.
This is a group with free therapy exercises for people with aphasia.

Find a support group for people with aphasia in your area.

1. Go to aphasia.org
2. Click on: I have aphasia
3. Click on: I need support/therapy
4. Under the subtitle: <u>So how can a speech-language pathologist help me?</u> There is a link in blue that says: <u>Click here to find a support group.</u> Click on it.
5. Click on the first two boxes: Aphasia Centers and Programs and Aphasia Communication Groups.
6. Type in how many miles you are able to travel and your zip code and click <u>submit</u>
7. Call the number of the first support group listed and ask when they have meetings.

"When are your support groups for people with aphasia?"

Date:_____

Time:_____

Location:_____

Other Resources:

STAR Workbook I:

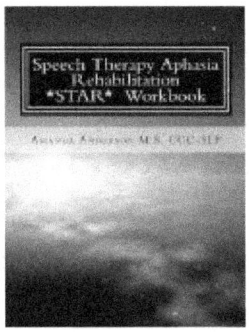

Expressive language

STAR Workbook II

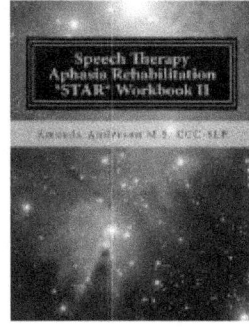

Receptive language

STAR Workbook III

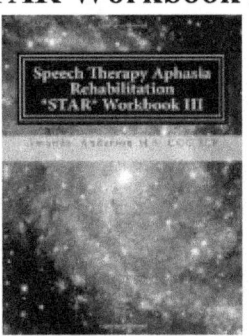

Descriptive language

ARC Guide

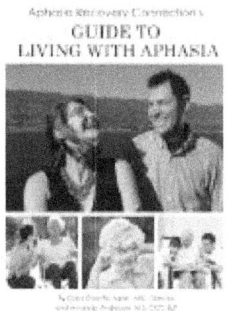

Guide to Living with Aphasia

Go to amazon.com search for "aphasia workbooks"